REBOUND

Redemption from Cancer
Journey of Life

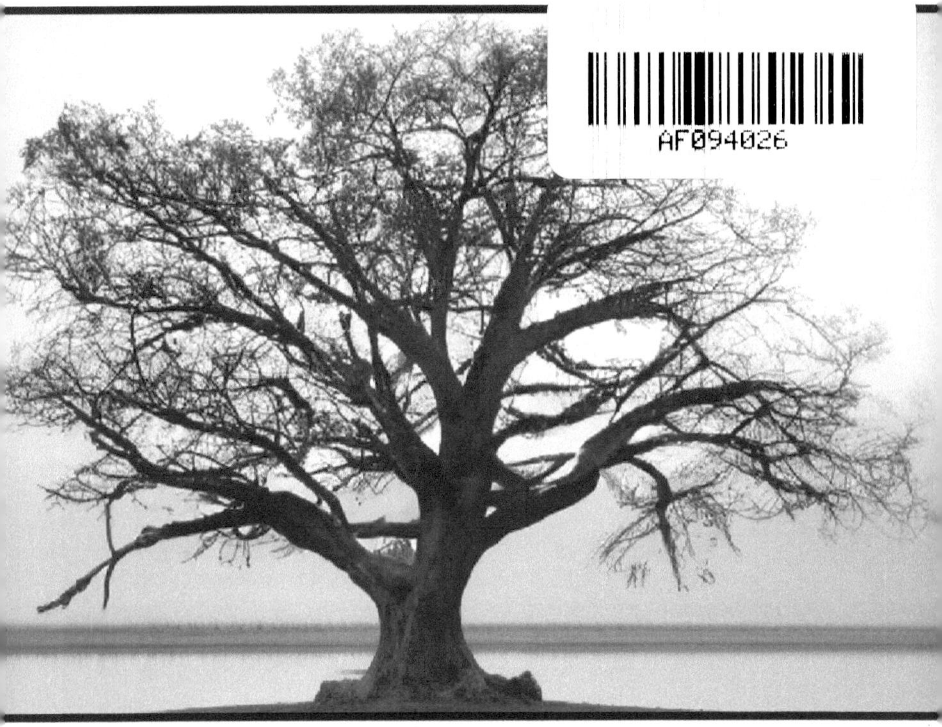

SUBHASH SETHI

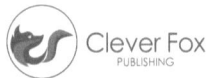
Clever Fox
PUBLISHING

CLEVER FOX PUBLISHING
Chennai, India

Published by CLEVER FOX PUBLISHING 2024
Copyright © SUBHASH SETHI 2024

All Rights Reserved.
PAPERBACK ISBN: 978-93-56483-57-6
HARDBACK ISBN: 978-93-56488-55-7

This book has been published with all reasonable efforts taken to make the material error-free after the consent of the author. No part of this book shall be used, reproduced in any manner whatsoever without written permission from the author, except in the case of brief quotations embodied in critical articles and reviews.

The Author of this book is solely responsible and liable for
its content including but not limited to the views, representations, descriptions, statements, information, opinions and references ["Content"]. The Content of this book shall not constitute or be construed or deemed to reflect the opinion or expression of the Publisher or Editor. Neither the Publisher nor Editor endorse or approve the Content of this book or guarantee the reliability,
accuracy or completeness of the Content published herein
and do not make any representations or warranties of any kind, express or implied, including but not limited to the implied
warranties of merchantability, fitness for a particular purpose.
The Publisher and Editor shall not be liable whatsoever for
any errors, omissions, whether such errors or omissions result from negligence, accident, or any other cause or claims for loss or damages of any kind, including without limitation, indirect or consequential loss or damage arising out of use, inability to use, or about the reliability, accuracy or sufficiency of the information contained in this book.

A tale of passion and resilience

DISCLAIMER

The book is an effort to put forward the author's life experiences during various stages of his cancer treatment and the lessons he has derived from it. It does not intend to preach life lessons like any other book on self-development.

The book also does not limit the reader to believing that these are the only lessons that can be learned during and after the disease. Different patients might surely come up with different experiences. The author desires that the reader gain the knowledge that can have a positive impact on their well-being. It also tries to act as a guide for people undergoing similar conditions.

The book also does not intend to hurt any professional, religious or regional sentiments and the author does not endorse any motive or bias.

The book is solely written with the intention of creating awareness of cancer and gaining knowledge and inspiration from the life lessons of Subhash Sethi.

THE INSCRIPTION

Rebound truly touched my heart with the author's unwavering spirit and belief in the power of hope. He shows us that cancer is not just a disease to be fought but an opportunity for personal growth and transformation. Through his own journey, he shares valuable lessons about self-care, the importance of a strong support network, and the significance of embracing each day as a gift. It serves as a guiding light for those diagnosed with cancer, their loved ones, and anyone seeking inspiration and hope in the face of adversity.

I wholeheartedly recommend *Rebound* to anyone touched by cancer or seeking a transformative story of resilience. Prepare to be moved, enlightened, and empowered as you embark on this remarkable journey with the author. His words will leave an everlasting imprint on your soul and remind you of the power of the human spirit to overcome even the greatest challenges.

– Dr. Lal Thanhawla, Former Chief Minister of Mizoram

Cancer patients find themselves feeling confused and adrift after a diagnosis. They struggle to understand the medical jargon while dealing with emotional issues and uncertainty. Even cancer treatment becomes a difficult and often challenging experience. Mr. Sethi has beautifully described all these in his book *Rebound* after getting cured of a rare type of throat cancer. He has described life's most difficult challenges in fighting cancer to make it a readable and comprehensive guide for patients, their families, and people associated in such a manner that it can easily be called 'a book on wellness strategies.' This book is a source of good information and patients at any stage of cancer will find it tremendously useful because it can help them cope more effectively.

I wish him good health and happiness.

– Sushmita Sen, Bollywood Star

Cancer treatment presents a challenging journey, demanding immense strength, resilience, and determination. Just as sportsperson harness discipline to conquer hurdles and surpass their limits, individuals facing cancer can draw upon the same fortitude to navigate the physical, emotional, and mental hurdles. Discipline in cancer treatment extend to embracing self-care practices such as maintaining a healthy lifestyle, proper nutrition, regular exercise, and adequate rest.

In the book *Rebound,* the author shares a compelling account of how adhering to medical protocols and treatment plans with unwavering sincerity led to a full recovery from a rare type of cancer. This story serves as a powerful testament to the significance of discipline in cancer treatment for better outcomes.

Bhaichung Bhutia, Former International Football Player

THE INSCRIPTION

In this book, he intimately shares with us his journey so that we need not fear, we learn to cope and how best to recover. He narrates the importance of deep familial love and support and regales us with stories of his relatives and close friends who came to surround him with love, care and affection. His gentle chiding of those doctors or nurses who have become so immune to suffering given the number of medical cases they see on a daily basis, that they forget each patient is a unique individual who needs emotional support, kind words and gentle treatment when confronted by this disease. In this book, he also tells us of the importance of the right diet to avoid feeding the beast with sugar and to have the right environment to recuperate. He speaks of the importance of his religious faith and his abiding hope. I commend you for this book because it's a story of fostering correct thought, correct action correct company and support in the face of human adversity, which is inevitable.

– **Jimmy Yim, Chairman, Drew & Napier LLC**

Rebound is an extremely engaging narration, each of its chapter shares a life experience which connects very well with the audience and offers a lot to learn. The learning and mantras that have been shared are a delight to read. It is a powerful testament to the unwavering determination that resides within each one of us, waiting to be awakened in the face of adversity. This book is a beacon of hope and strength for anyone facing this formidable disease. It is an incredible story of the author who faced the terrifying diagnosis head-on and refused to succumb to despair. It offers a roadmap to harness one's inner strength and find solace amidst the turmoil. *Rebound* has the ability to empower and uplift the reader.

– **T. V. Narendran, MD, Tata Steel Limited**

This book is a first-hand account of author's experience with cancer. Mr. Subhash Sethi has been my patient for a decade. He shares his personal journey through diagnosis, treatment, and ultimately, remission. This book provides a glimpse into the physical, emotional, and mental toll that a diagnosis of malignancy can take on a person and their loved ones.

I was struck by author's honesty and vulnerability in sharing his story in this book. He does not shy away from the difficult parts of his journey, but rather, he confronts them head-on. His courage and resilience in the face of such adversity are truly inspiring. While this book is a personal account, it also sheds light on the broader issues surrounding cancer treatment. The author touches on the importance of a strong support system, particularly family support, and the challenges of navigating the healthcare system.

I believe that this book will be a valuable resource for anyone who is going through the same ordeal, whether as a patient or a caregiver. It provides a unique perspective that can only come from someone who has lived through the experience. I hope that this book will serve as a source of comfort and inspiration for those who are currently passing through a similar phase in life.

– **Dr. Bijay Patni, Renowned Physician in Kolkata**

THE INSCRIPTION

I was so happy to hear how bravely he fought cancer and came out fully recovered. I was very delighted when he told me that he had compiled a book on his battle to fight cancer. I really admire how he has shared his journey from detection to recovery and tried to inspire people by stating the facts surrounding cancer, the adversities he faced during that period and how he overcame them with the help and support of his family and close friends. This step is very inspirational and motivational as it would help and give strength to a lot of people to stay positive and fight the battle and never give up or lose hope.

– Dr. Kuldeep Jain, District Judge. Sarangpur, Madhya Pradesh

---

Cancer is certainly a dreadful disease and its manifestation has increased over the last few decades. The book *Rebound* by Mr. Subhash Sethi has captivated my attention with the detailing he has done about being diagnosed with a rare form of cancer and his determination to overthrow his nemesis. His frank remarks on the changing trends in medical treatment becoming more mechanical than human are indeed concerning. He has presented very good information in this book that will be helpful to not only cancer patients, survivors, and their families but every reader to gain knowledge and referring it to anybody if ever challenged.

– Ashok Patni, Chairman, Wonder Cement

Rebound, as the name suggests, is about resilience in the face of life-threatening adversity. The book offers a glimpse into the mind of the person and thoughts that takeover when one discovers the illness and it suggests practical steps that can help stay positive. No one is ever prepared for cancer and often finds oneself in lonely and uncharted territory in the battle with the disease. *Rebound* serves as a guidebook not just for patients but also for friends and family emphasising the role of a robust support system towards meaningful recovery. All this is in a well-structured format sprinkled with the personal experiences of a successful cancer survivor.

– Harsh Goenka, Chairman, RPG Enterprises

Rebound nonchalantly achieves what it sets out to do. The book stretches out a hand to hold for someone recently diagnosed with cancer or undergoing treatment for it, with anxieties and unanswered questions pent up inside him or her. Subhash Sethi relives his emotional turmoil through various stages of his tryst with the disease in painstaking detail, right from the inconclusive biopsy reports to his trepidations when chemotherapy begins. He writes about his changing attitude towards the disease as months pass and treatment progresses and, of course, about the unflinching support of his extended family. The author professes the need for an environment of positivity for people fighting cancer along with proper treatment, not from the pulpit but sitting at the bedside with an arm around the patient's shoulder.

– Dr. Rupali Basu, Managing Director & CEO, Woodlands Multispeciality Hospital, Kolkata

---

Rebound is a reminder that while cancer may be a formidable opponent, nothing can withstand the power of holistic healing. It captures how a positive mindset, supportive environment, and healthy lifestyle can transform the journey from diagnosis to recovery.

**– Chandrajit Banerjee, Director General,
Confederation of Indian Industry (CII)**

Rebound is a nonfictional account of an industrialist-turned-patient diagnosed with cancer, as well as his emotional and physical trials through that experience. Dealing with uncertainty often turns out to be messier than we anticipate and those who are not prepared or who have the wrong expectations give up too quickly. Mr. Sethi's tale provides rare insight into human emotions and experiences with inspiration derived from his treatment. As a physician working and forever learning the art of cancer care, I gained insight into the patient experience which can be difficult to account for in the bustle of hospitals and the internal challenges that often come with these experiences. This book empathetically motivates us to value what we should treasure most in the world—our health.

**– Dr. S K Sogani, Senior Consultant (Neurology),
Apollo Hospital, New Delhi**

What makes *Rebound* special is the power of believing in your mission when you're trying to get yourself treated and cured of a difficult ailment called cancer. This book is a great reminder of what it takes to fight invisible intruders. Subhash Sethi is proof that it's possible to pick the hardest problems and tackle them effectively through willpower, ingenuity and mental strength. By telling the story of his own life, he inspires others not to give up, not to succumb and to push through all over again. It's more than a book—it is a reference manual for cancer patients.

– Mr. Shailendra Jain, CEO & Founder, Abaqus Inc., USA

Rebound effectively portrays the idea that our most remarkable achievements can only be reached when we wholeheartedly embrace challenges and embark on a journey fuelled by resilience. The profound narrative, spanning from the initial cancer detection to the triumphant recovery of the author, serves as a powerful inspiration. With meticulous attention to detail, he sparks hope and rejuvenates our spirits, highlighting the vital importance of perseverance in the face of adversity. Moreover, he emphasize the profound significance of family values and the adoption of healthy practice as indispensable pillars for cultivating a well-balanced lifestyle.

– Atul Pandey IRS, Additional Commissioner Income Tax

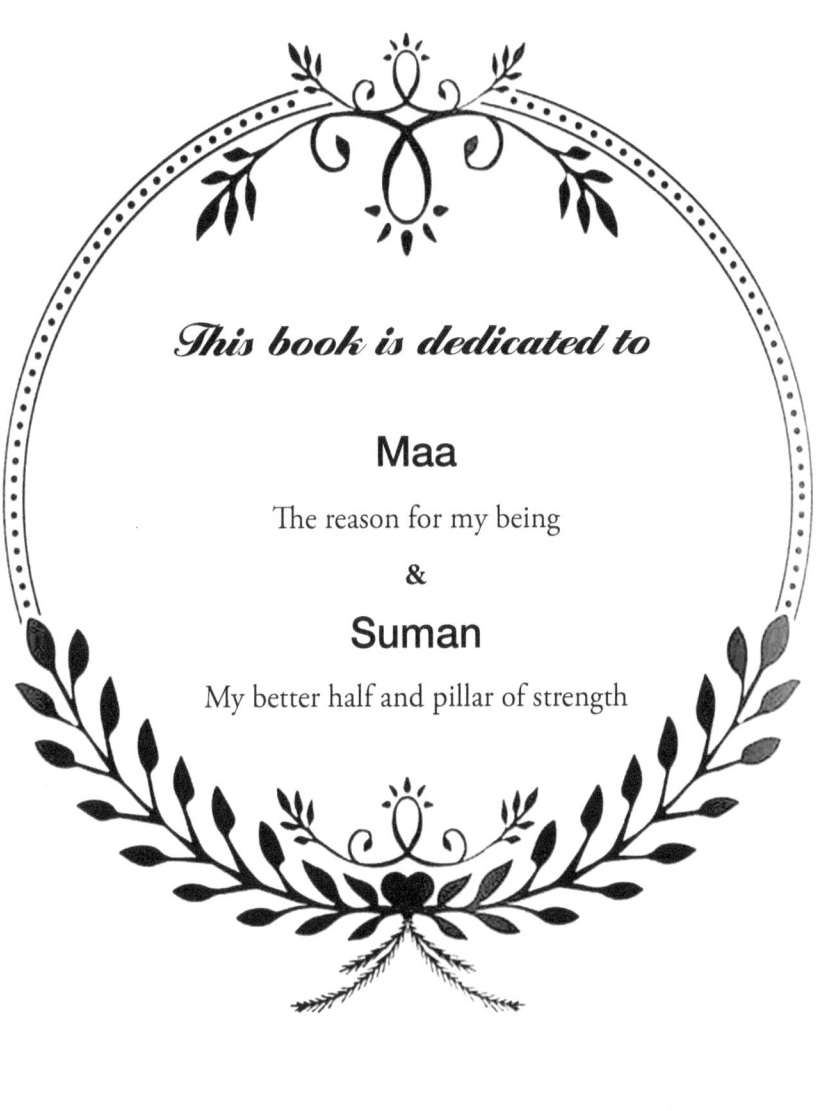

This book is dedicated to

Maa

The reason for my being

&

Suman

My better half and pillar of strength

CONTENTS

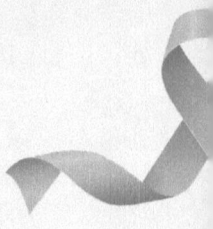

The Inscription v
About The Book xvii
About The Author xix
Foreword xxi
Acknowledgement xxiii
Introduction xxvii

PHASE 1: Before Cancer 1

1 Early Memories — 2

2 The Beginning of Becoming — 7

3 The Urge to Grow — 14

4 The Times That Are Now — 17

CONTENTS

PHASE 2: The Detection 25

5 Early Symptoms   26

6 The Investigation   32

7 The Findings   39

8 The Beginning of Treatment   48

9 Pillars of Strength   73

PHASE 3: Recovery 85

10 The Road to Recovery   86

11 Emerging out of Umbra   96

12 Back to the City of Joy   104

13 Moments to Cherish   107

14 Invaluable Life Lessons   114

15 Sailing to Health   127

16 Solitude Connects You With yourself   141

17 The Inspiration	157
18 My Heartfelt Message	167
19 The Viewpoints	171

Frequently Asked Questions (FAQs) *179*
Cancer Etiquette *188*
References *192*
Inspire *195*

ABOUT THE BOOK

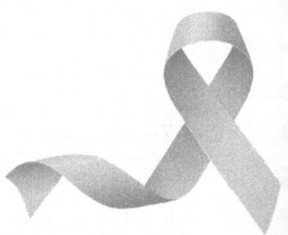

This book seeks to inspire readers by shedding light on facts surrounding cancer and providing practical life lessons from my valuable learning and experiences. It primarily chronicles my personal journey of fighting against cancer and finding recovery. In different chapters, I share insights from detection to treatment and recount my own experiences. A strong believer in destiny, one of the key lessons I learned is that destiny sets the direction and destination of our lives. I encourage readers not to dwell on the past or worry about the uncertain future, but to embrace the present and find joy in the moment.

Expressing gratitude and appreciating the support of family and friends during life's ups and downs is a central theme in this book. It emphasizes finding happiness and positivity in life's little gifts. With a positive mindset and unwavering self-belief, one can overcome any adversity, including a formidable disease like cancer.

The chapters in this book provide insights into cancer cells and its causes, advocating for a healthy lifestyle to safeguard against this lethal disorder. It also reminds us that certain things in life are beyond our control, as evidenced during the COVID pandemic. Yet, staying positive is crucial in not giving up, accepting problems as they come, and seeking multiple opinions from specialists before proceeding with treatment and recovery.

This book also delves into revisiting human traits during moments of solitude and cultivating gratitude for the blessings we often take for granted. It underscores the importance of fostering a positive mindset to create a better world.

My challenging journey from diagnosis to treatment has taught me profound life lessons and a deeper understanding of life's intricacies. It encourages readers to purposefully slow down and reflect on life's numerous facets.

I genuinely hope that the valuable lessons shared in this book will impact lives, bring hope, and instill positivity in the hearts of its readers.

ABOUT THE AUTHOR

SUBHASH SETHI

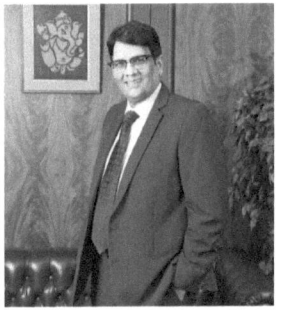

Subhash Sethi is the chairman of SPML Infra Limited, a publicly listed infrastructure development company in India. For almost five decades, he has worked relentlessly with an inspirational mission to create sustainable value and wealth for the country.

Under his leadership, SPML Infra has gone on to establish itself as one of the leading engineering and infrastructure development organizations in India with over 650 completed projects in the domain of water, power, sanitation, the environment, and civil infrastructure.

Armed with business education, quick wits and a firm belief in his potential, Sethi crafted a success story by leading from the front and making his company build sustainable infrastructure through exemplary engineering and execution capabilities and delivering safe and clean drinking water to about 50 million people of India every day.

He is also recognized as an industry spokesperson and represents industry associations like CII, Indian Chamber of Commerce, etc. as their Committee Chairman. His valuable contributions towards the development of sustainable infrastructure in India have been widely recognized and he has received several prestigious awards and accolades from industry bodies and institutions including the International Economic Times Asian Business Leaders Award.

FOREWORD

It is with great pleasure and admiration that I write this foreword for Subhash's book, which chronicles his journey towards embracing and managing cancer.

Over the past 9-10 years, my team and I have worked with several cancer patients from around the world, some early-stage, some end-stage, and some end-of-life. Among them are those whose journeys stand out as truly inspiring, and Subhash's journey is one of them.

As you read through the pages of this book, you will gain insight into the incredible strength, commitment, humility, discipline, optimism, and consistency that Subhash possessed in order to overcome a disease that can be overwhelming to even the bravest of souls. While my team and I can guide individuals on how nutrition, emotional health, movement and activity, sleep, and lifestyle can positively impact the progression of the disease, the most important work of putting knowledge into action must be done by the individual themselves. And that is what sets Subhash apart.

In my decade-long practice in integrative and lifestyle medicine, I have yet to see two cancer patients, despite having the same type of cancer, following the same protocol, taking the same medications, and so on, have the same outcomes. Every cancer patient's journey is unique and different, and do you know what creates this difference? The patient himself! His attitude, mindset, belief, faith, perception of the treatment, his body's intelligence, and the disease create different outcomes.

Subhash's inspiring story is a testament to the power of an integrative approach to cancer using the best of medicine and lifestyle, a strong mindset, and personalized care.

This book is not only an inspiration for individuals with cancer but for everyone. Subhash's life lessons, learnings, and unlearning will leave a lasting impact on all who read. It is a legacy for generations to come.

Subhash, I wish you all the success with this book and I intend the best of health and life for you from my heart.

It was an honor to partner with you on your journey and I am grateful to be able to put these words down for all your readers.

With love and gratitude,

– Luke Coutinho
Expert Nutritionist, Holistic & Wellness Coach

ACKNOWLEDGEMENT

The idea of writing this book is to share my experience with a rare type of cancer for which I received successful treatment. I have shared my learning about treatment and important aspects of cancer in this book in a profound way to turn life-threatening challenges into attainments. It contains practical prescriptions for successfully meeting some of life's most difficult setbacks.

Spoken words are meant to have long-lasting effects and I have experienced it in a most striking and motivating manner. "Beta, tune itni pariksha paas ki hai, ye bhi karlega (Son, you have passed several exams, you will also pass this)." These words coming from Maa (my mother) worked like a booster dose. After the cancer was detected, I was very concerned and stressed. When my mother saw me, she asked what happened.

Before I could say anything, my wife, Suman replied saying, "Ek badi pariksha hai Maa (Mummy, it's a big exam)." Upon hearing the word "pariksha (exam)", she had responded. I just cannot describe the new energy that ran into me after hearing my mother saying the lines and I told my inner self that I have the blessings of my mother and no matter what the situation comes, I will be victorious. I am extremely indebted to my mother for making me realise that I can win over any adversity.

I would like to express my deepest gratitude to my wife, Suman Sethi, who has been standing with me in all situations after my marriage to her.

My love and affection go beyond words for both my sons, Harsh and Abhinandan. I must commend their untiring and determined efforts in finding the best possible treatment for me while keeping the smile on their faces to make me feel comfortable. Also to my adorable daughter, Roshni, for taking care of me with the utmost affection, empathy and care. The dedicated support of my daughters-in-law Shilpa and Priyanshi is beyond description.

My elder brother, Anil Sethi, younger brother, Sushil Sethi and my sister Rajul were very disturbed after knowing about my ailment and have given me tremendous moral and mental support which I will always be grateful for. Preeti Bhabi was concerned and caring about my health and well-being. Sushil's wife, Sandhya Sethi, my nephew, Rishabh and his wife, Aanchal have made extraordinary efforts for my peaceful and comfortable stay in Delhi.

My great appreciation to my niece, Dr. Noopur Jain and her husband, Dr. Ankit Jain, for taking good care of me and carefully managing all my needs during the entire period of my treatment in Delhi despite the COVID pandemic which was at its peak.

I also appreciate the ardent support and concerns of all my other family members, my in-laws, my friends, business colleagues, my son's in-laws, nephews, and nieces.

ACKNOWLEDGEMENT

It would be incomplete if I did not talk about Ashok Patni Ji, Suresh Patni Ji and Vimal Patni Ji, C.P Kothari Ji, D. P. Kothari Ji, Sunil Kothari and Mrs. Neeta Boochra for visiting me despite their busy schedules and they also frequently called up for regular updates.

I would like to express my deep gratitude to Dr. Ashok Vaid for guiding me to the right treatment and recovery. I would also like to express my heartfelt thanks to Dr. S. K. Sogani, Dr. Sanjay Jain, Dr. Bijay Patni, Dr. Balram Prasad, Dr. Deepak Sarin, Dr. Ankur Bahl, Dr. Roshan Dixit, Dr. Manju Sengar, Dr. Anita Borges, Mr. Luke Coutinho (Holistic & Wellness Coach), Dr. Jayesh, Dr. Colin Phipps Diong and Dr. Akhil Chopra of Mount Elizabeth Hospital, Singapore, Dr. Arushi Khurana of Mayo Clinic, USA and of course, Dr. Nitin Sood, who had done my final PET Scan and declared me free of disease. My appreciation to all the nursing and support staff in Medanta Hospital who treated me with great care and respect.

I wish to express my deepest gratitude to my Guru Ji for his pious blessings that have given me immense spiritual and mental support during the most difficult days of my life and in coming out of this frightening disease.

My earnest thanks to my cherished friends, Kamal Surana, Pawan Patni, Nirmal Kothari and Suresh Patni. My special thanks to S. K. Tulsiyan ji for his concern and prayers for my speedy recovery.

I would also like to thank Mr. Lalit Hundlani, Mr. Satadal Lahiri and of course Tariq Siddiqui for helping me write this book. I would also like to express my thanks and appreciation to all members of SPML Infra and Group Companies for their prayers and support during my treatment.

I firmly believe that this book will provide a deep understanding of cancer and my experience of how to combat it successfully.

My sincere and special thanks to all the readers of this book!

– Subhash Sethi

INTRODUCTION

"There is nothing certain but the uncertain."

– Anonymous

I have heard and believed that time and tide wait for none. Time does not care about hierarchy, position or honour. It has its own way to trouble and teach, warn and welcome and hurt and heal. We are paltry beings who, more often than not tend to disregard the power of time. People learn valuable lessons from various phases of life through joy, agony and emotional upheavals. As I rose through the torrents of time after being diagnosed and treated for cancer, I, too, have learned immensely about life through life itself.

This is not only a survivor's tale but a sharing of lessons that I have picked up in the process, which I believe, is something that we should know but, of course, without going through the tumultuous stages of cancer or any other peril.

I have had a strong will since my childhood. It is not that I was born with a silver spoon but I do consider myself privileged. I had a decent upbringing, a good education, a visionary father, a loving mother, three siblings and other-worldly facilities such as an electric fan, a landline phone, etc. that we often take for granted. I had friends to play with and dreams that looked possible to achieve.

Even after climbing the ladder of success, life had yet another twist that I never expected. I faced adversity while growing up and creating a world of my own by re-enforcing my father's dream. I started my adventurous journey under the guidance of my visionary father and encountered hurdles and challenges. But I was never really prepared for a bigger challenge.

No school, college, or institution ever teaches us about coping with the fear of death. Though it is inevitable, it has a defined process. It tells us how we should make honest efforts to live a fulfilling life.

When I write about this, the following lines from Langston Hughes's poem come to mind:

> "Life is for the living.
>
> Death is for the dead.
>
> Let life be like music.
>
> And death a note unsaid."

It is more important to know, understand and appreciate the values and goodness of life. We fail to notice and acknowledge that we are privileged. We are privileged to have a lot of things that we often take for granted. Nature, relationships, happiness, being loved and respected, the feelings of gratitude, appreciation, devotion, hope, love and the ability to discover and re-discover are all priceless treasures.

INTRODUCTION

One of the greatest beliefs that I have fostered since childhood is that God always does the best for us in His own majestic way. The strong faith that my family, my father especially fostered has created a strong belief system in me and my brothers. I have always believed that destiny is fixed for everyone. No matter what comes your way, your destiny will always rule your direction. There were times when I came across challenges that looked insurmountable. However, my belief and strong faith in destiny helped me overcome such situations.

I am a risk-taker. I have developed the nerve to laugh in the face of adversity and am always prepared to take challenges head-on. People sometimes contact me for solutions and I gladly help them. I do not advocate giving unsolicited advice even if someone values my opinion or is facing the same problem as me. Unwarranted advice and opinions are mental burdens. Encouragement and motivation work well in such situations.

Every life has an inherent story but the underlying fact is that God has gifted us with a wonderful life. We are not destined to live forever but we should enjoy every moment we have. That is the most important and greatest tribute that we can pay to our creator.

My idea for this book is to share the lessons I have learned through this phase of life and I wish to help each reader learn from these universal lessons.

I have tried to list out all possible references that patients might need during or after the treatment of severe diseases. Some references to doctors, clinics, labs, medicines, food and habits have been incorporated to provide people with the proper knowledge to combat and overcome a disease like cancer.

The message is clear! Anyone can get infected with a life-threatening disease. However, God has given us the inherent power to overcome and heal. Medical science is advancing at a rapid pace and today, a disease like cancer can be effectively treated and cured. God forbid, if one of you is diagnosed with cancer, keep faith that you can surely overcome it.

PHASE 1

BEFORE CANCER

EARLY MEMORIES

Guwahati had been the starting point of my journey. My visionary father, Punam Chand Sethi Ji, had incorporated my siblings and myself into modest but developing water pump company on the testing grounds. Initially, the escalating insurgency of various political and social factions in Assam had a negative impact on the industry.

Despite difficult times, my father was a resourceful and righteous businessman. Not only he was full of ideas; but he was also a man of action. He had never compromised with his principles and provided the best quality products and services to all his customers. This attribute had always made him endearing to everybody and also brought in more business. Despite being fully engaged in his business venture, he was a devout family man who spent quality time with the family and was also available for community welfare services.

I had a strong belief in destiny, and this is what I consider to be the most outstanding attribute that I learned from my father. This belief never allowed him to feel saddened, overwhelmed or disturbed under any circumstance and I derived this confidence and belief from him that God will always lead us to the right path.

EARLY MEMORIES

His helpful and humble nature along with his strong value system always won him respect and reverence from his friends and peers as well as from his clients and competitors. As his son, I feel blessed and proud to have inherited his qualities and abilities to help me conquer any situation in life.

My vision, however, had gone beyond the water pump business. I wanted to venture into bigger grounds and started strengthening my network and knowledge in the realm of water treatment. We started bidding for smaller projects, passionately pursued my ideas and succeeded in winning a few small water projects. I had support from my brothers who strengthened my will to propel the company to higher echelons. My elder brother, Anil Sethi, soon migrated to Bangalore and my younger brother, Sushil Sethi, to Delhi to spread the organization's name far and wide while I chose to settle in Calcutta (now Kolkata), the city of joy.

Water business has been our forte for almost five decades now.

On a professional front, we were rising rapidly but we had to stabilize our personal lives. My elder brother Anil Sethi, who is 4 years older than me, had been married to Preeti Bhabi and my parents were in search of the right match for me.

When it came to me, my parents were aware of my mental framework, likes, and dislikes and most importantly, my aspirations in life. They had kept these in their list of priorities while selecting my life partner Suman, to whom I got married on the 10th of July in 1980. Though my wife is 5 years younger than me, she has been more of a friend and supported me like a rock through testing times. I will be forever grateful to her for making my life beautiful. She has always stood by me during times that were rough and stormy to help me bounce back. She had always reminded me of the dictum that defeat is never declared when you fall down; it is announced only if you refuse to get up. She has also time and again emphasized, like my parents, that it is far more honorable to fail than to cheat.

Over the years I have become the proud father of three precious children. My daughter, Roshni Jain, the eldest of siblings, lives in Bengaluru and is a prominent jewellery designer and licensed RTT therapist. Harshvardhan (Harsh) Sethi, who is the eldest of my sons, is presently the MD and director of our group of companies and looks after all international business ventures. Abhinandan Sethi, my younger son is the executive director of SPML Infra Limited, heading all the day-to-day activities of the company. It is a joy to be with my children and grandchildren whenever we come together to spend quality and blissful times.

In my early days, I remember taking up a very challenging project of building water supply infrastructure in Lunglei, Mizoram. Here drinking water had to be taken to the habitats situated at the top of a hill at a height of 880 metres above ground level. The height was a major issue and most people would prefer to split the climb for safety measures.

It was a very difficult task to laying pipelines in the hilly terrain. But with grit and resilience, we decided to take the water on a single inclination from ground level to the top. It was a huge risk as a rupture in the pipeline would not only inundate the whole area but also cause severe casualties. Hence, before the commissioning we had managed to convince the government to vacate the adjoining villages as a safety measure.

The seamless and trouble-free commissioning of the system brought great joy to me, my family and people all around for achieving something unthinkable. The courage to take a risk had paid off. We had won against heavy odds and this project had gone on to be a trendsetter for more such projects in the future and the memories of it are still etched in my mind even after 40 years.

> Challenges and successes all through my life journey have positive manifestations.

Through unrelenting hard work and passionate pursuits, our company received admiration as we built numerous prestigious projects in water supply, wastewater treatment, power transmission & distribution, and other projects. The Chief Minister of Mizoram, Mr. Lal Thanhawla and the implementing agencies highly appreciated our commitment and extraordinary efforts with a qualitative and strategic approach. They also commended us for our steady growth and relentless pursuit of excellence. Soon, the media and statisticians started following our progress and appreciating our development.

There have been challenges and successes throughout my life and it has all the ingredients for me to believe that life has been kind to me with all positive manifestations. However, life doesn't hold any prototypes and this realization about the true meaning of life came to me through one of the toughest examinations that I had to go through. The test of my courage was yet to come.

However, when given the choice of opting for a city to spend the most difficult sessions of my life—my cancer treatment—I selected Delhi for a meaningful reason. I will reveal the reason in the later chapters and I am sure readers will resonate with the dominance attached to the selection.

THE BEGINNING OF BECOMING

I remember a line I read in Michelle Obama's book, *Becoming* where she writes, "The lesson being that in life you control what you can."

I believe that if you wish to make your life purposeful, you can control it to achieve what you wish. It is important that you know that I consider myself to be an ordinary man. I have no special powers and if I can sail through the dark storms of cancer, others also can.

I was born into a family of freedom fighters in Ladnun, the *tehsil* (sub division) of the Nagaur district in Rajasthan. This town is renowned for its religious beliefs and culture as it is the birthplace of the sacred Jain Aacharya, Tulsi. Our ancestral house was a *haveli (mansion)* and a prominent building in the area. My paternal grandfather, Keshri Chand Sethi ji was a famous and revered person, had many contacts due to his booming business in bullion trading.

Ladnun has a complex of Jain temples that were found by the archeologists while excavating and as per the inscription found on one of the doors of the temple, it was constructed in the year 1136. Ladnun is also home to the Jain Vishva Bharati University and other old temples of religious and architectural importance. It is a prominent pilgrimage spot for people from the Jain community. Additionally, there are many places of religious and scenic significance in close proximity, drawing tourists and pilgrims from all over the world. Ladnun is also known for its exquisite cotton sarees which have always found interested customers from all over.

Though I was very young during my days in Ladnun, I remember the respect that our family received from people and the selfless love and camaraderie that existed everywhere. During the summer months, I also remember the extreme temperatures and frequent sand storms that we had to encounter.

It was a happy childhood for me and my brothers. We loved to play outdoors with the other children and would often be scolded for spending so much time under the scorching sun. Due to the family's strong religious beliefs, we have been instilled with a deep faith in God and various spiritual aspects of life. I have always admired my parent's deep conviction in God and the goodness in life itself.

Shifting Base:

My father, Punam Chand Sethi ji, was an outgoing person and wanted to start a business that would attract global acclaim. His numerous contacts and strong connections helped him get an opportunity in water pumps which he started in Guwahati, Assam. In 1967, my family moved from the western part of India to the northeast, where we had to adapt to a completely different culture, food, lifestyle, climate, linguistic patterns, geography and demography. The family had responded to the challenge willingly.

THE BEGINNING OF BECOMING

I was admitted to L.O.G. Hindi School in Guwahati, one of the oldest schools in a fancy bazaar area, where I also completed my board examination with fairly good marks. It was one of the few Hindi medium schools in Assam. My father's immense regard for traditional values made him choose this school since it imparted a lot of behavioral-based teachings. The school used to be a center for not only academic learning but also self-development as well. There used to be countless life lessons taught in school that are still applicable even today.

There was also a unique system in the school to impart lessons through storytelling. I remember my English and Mathematics teacher, Late Mahesh Jha, who was a kind-hearted person always ready to motivate us to think out of the box and plan to achieve greater goals in life. This method of education is highly impactful since moral, social, practical developmental and scientific lessons can be imparted very easily.

Our teachers, therefore, always tried to impart important lessons by sharing stories of Akbar and Birbal. The central character, Birbal was the advisor and main commander of the army in the court of the emperor, Akbar. When in a dilemma, the emperor, generally seek advice from the quick-witted Birbal for instant solutions.

I am tempted to share one such moral story about Akbar and Birbal. There is a famous story on the topic of everything happening for the good. I hope you like it as there is an embedded message that in our lives, some incidents happen. We may not like it at that time but, mostly, they prove to be good for us.

One day, Akbar and Birbal went hunting in the forest. Blood was flowing from a cut on Akbar's finger.

Birbal told the king, "Do not worry. God does what he does only for the good. Have faith."

Akbar was so disturbed by the pain that when he heard Birbal's statement, he became angry. Hence, he ordered that Birbal be imprisoned immediately. Following the order of the king, the soldiers immediately arrested Birbal and put him in jail.

> "Do not worry, God does what he does, for good only, have faith"

The next day, the king went hunting deep in the forest but somehow got separated from his troops. He was apprehended by a group of cannibals while wondering around looking for a way out. They took him to their leader and started preparing to sacrifice him to their divine. Seeing Akbar's slit finger, the head priest of the cannibals announced that since he was wounded, his sacrifice could not be accepted.

They freed him and Akbar was found by his soldiers and returned to the palace. He remembered Birbal's words and realized his mistake. He got him free and hugged him. Akbar told him about the incident and asked, "If I cut my finger, then God saved my life. But what good came out of me sending you to prison?"

Birbal smiled and said, "Had you not put me in prison, I would have been with you and they would have sacrificed me in your place. Therefore, whatever God does, it is only for good."

Many factors are sometimes overlooked and taken for granted. However, these are the truths that life has presented to us and it is good if we follow them in life. The moral of this story has worked miraculously for me.

I still remember a few stories with underlying messages that were told to me during my student days. While I was in the hospital room during my chemotherapy, I used to remember those stories during my time of solitude and they would bring smile on my face. Those stories were meaningful and had a deep impact on me and I still cherish them. The quick-wittedness and analytical traits that are inherent in me can partly be attributed to those stories.

Additionally, there was a session in our school that inculcated the art of listening and observing which has helped me to this date. Many times, we get overwhelmed with our mundane lives and tend to overlook or ignore some meaningful messages that may impact our thinking process. There have been people who have time and again come to me to talk about their woes in life. Some had family problems; some had financial issues; some had problems related to health; and some had other problems that they were unable to explain to anyone. I did exactly what I have seen my father do in such situations. He never judged, ridiculed, or advised anyone as to how he would have handled their situation. He just listened

> As a student, I learned the art of listening and observing in my school that has helped me tremendously.

to them attentively. People want someone to listen to them and I believe that patiently listening is itself an art. This quality makes you endearing to people.

I would love to mention here that many employees in our company are from our ancestral place. They have been with us for many years and have always been treated like members of a big family. They have been given the respect and concern that they deserve and they too have reciprocated it time and again with their loyalty and faith. I have always had an emotional connection with them and have always cared to listen to them and understand each of them better. When I was away for treatment, I came to know that many people prayed and cried for me. They were clerks, drivers, gardeners, helpers and other staff members in my office apart from the senior officials who too shared their concerns.

It is important to observe even the smallest things in life. It is a joy to see my mother doing the small things that we generally take for granted. My mother also decoded the emotions on our faces and provided solutions to our concerns in no time. The power of observation of a human being is immense only if we try to put it into practice.

I remember one of the teachers in high school telling us an anecdote that urged us to observe small things that matter in a big way.

After World War II, Stalin's Soviet Russia went behind the iron curtain. It was a period when the affairs of Russia were not known to the rest of the world. The Russian news agencies simply proclaimed that there was nothing but prosperity with the Moscow markets overflowing with goods.

Two inquisitive journalists from London, Jack Colley and David Jones, decided to explore reality. Through various means, Jack managed to obtain a visa but David was unfortunate to have his papers rejected. So, they hatched a plan. Jack would travel to Russia and write back to David talking about the prosperity and all possible positives about Russia to escape the heavy scrutiny of the outgoing letters. It was decided between the two that if the lines were written in blue ink they were supposed to be taken to be the truth. However, if written in red ink, it would mean just the opposite.

A week later the letter came, it was written in blue about the prosperity of the people and the tremendous development Russia was going through. David believed in the contents of the letter since it was in blue, and he managed to send the contents to the news agencies around London. However, he missed noticing a small note at the end of the letter.

The note said, "The only thing that I could not find in the Moscow markets was red ink."

These lessons are unforgettable. During the toughest days of my life which were full of distress and dismay, when even my survival seemed to be at stake, I realized that they cheered us up.

THE URGE TO GROW

I recall my father's words, emphasizing that my actions would shape who I aspire to be and that the choices I make today will determine my future self. These lines have powered and inspired my journey from childhood to where I am today and all credit goes to him for instilling the importance of actions in life.

While I was a student, I used to read the success stories of famous personalities and how they combated adversities to make it to the top. This has inspired me to think about my career ahead of time. Even during schooling, I used to visit my father's business unit and try to learn the nuances of marketing and trade.

From humble beginnings in the water pump business, my father established a company known as 'Subhash Projects' which later became SPML Infra Limited, and this became a public listed company in 1983. After completing my graduation in Commerce from Guwahati University, along with my brother, Anil Sethi, I was inducted into the company in 1981. My father's mission was to create a global company and he had a long-term vision of providing clean drinking water facilities to people who lacked them. This inspired my brother and me to work hard and grow over the years.

I learned passion, dedication and selfless service from my father. Apart from developing a successful commercial business, throughout his life, he had a kind-hearted approach towards community development and the welfare of the economically weaker section of society. His demise in 2012 has created a big void in our family, that will always be difficult to fill.

While our business was flourishing, destiny had other plans for us. The political scenario in Assam was changing quite fast and the insurgency which was earlier confined to only certain pockets started spreading into the main cities. Due to constant disturbances, businesses in Assam started suffering heavily. Consequently, it became difficult for us to keep our business running in such a hostile condition.

The feeling of native residents vs outsiders was getting stronger. One day, my elder brother, Anil Sethi, was confronted by local people while out for work. They hurt his feelings by talking rudely to him. After a meaningful discussion with our father, all three brothers decided to relocate from Guwahati to other cities to develop our business.

There were many opportunities to expand our business and this prompted us to work cohesively to take the company to success and it soon started being noticed. Slowly, we developed our businesses and expanded the services from just water supply projects to wastewater treatment plants, power transmission and distribution and also sanitation projects. In a few years, our company was acknowledged among the best contracting firms in the country.

In our pursuit of excellence, there were, without a doubt, many challenges in the increasingly competitive arena of EPC projects. However, we never let the circumstances overwhelm us and continued our work with deep and dedicated focus. Due to our diligent approach, grit to compete, timely completion of projects, and sincere intent of not compromising on quality, we never faced dearth of orders. In fact, as soon as we relocated, our Delhi office secured a major order for water supply for the 1982 Asian Games. This job gave our credentials and prestige a huge boost. Simultaneously, we also secured some prestigious orders from Bengaluru and Kolkata.

THE TIMES THAT ARE NOW

There are times when you feel energetic and strong and there are times when you feel tired and exhausted. The hours you sleep definitely count in making you feel fresh to face the day ahead. However, whether you feel active and charged or sluggish and tired depends on the internal and external factors that determine your energy levels.

I remember attending a session of Sadhguru Shri Jaggi Vasudev in which he described that the level of energy in a person depends upon the food they eat, the water they drink, the air they breathe and the sunlight they receive. These things become the day-to-day energy that you experience. How alive and awake you are is reflective of how energetic you are. The ability to convert food, water, air and whatever other inputs go into your system will be different for different people.

I wanted to share my thoughts based on this context and my experiences. I wish to discuss the following aspects of life that I feel are important for people who are going through health issues and at times may feel helpless and overwhelmed by various complications that occur in the body.

There are always a few things that we should follow for the betterment of our health. Even if everything appears good and smooth in life, we should follow a disciplined way of living so that we can keep ourselves safe from infections and diseases.

Nowadays, life is full of speed and negativity. We find negative information published in newspapers and telecast throughout the day on various news channels. Many times, non-significant issues have been exaggerated to spread negative vibes. It is pertinent that one always remain positive and careful while living with this negativity. Here are some checkpoints that one should always review, even during good times, to ensure that sudden problems do not disturb the momentum.

1. All spiritual practices and meditations are fundamentally followed to make your energies more awake and keep you mentally calm.
2. Natural light is the strongest factor that controls our circadian rhythms. Your body knows that it's time to wake up and get going when it feels sunlight.
3. A brisk walk outside is the best way to keep your body recharged. As a bonus, exercise in the fresh air and sunshine boosts mood-lifting endorphins, the immune system and the metabolism.
4. Always keep yourself hydrated. Consuming an appropriate quantity of water keeps the body energized and healthy.
5. Caffeinated drinks give you a jolt of energy for some time but they can also cause you to feel even more tired when they wear off. It is a stimulant but doesn't have a long-lasting effect and can create dependency. Your stress levels tend to rise, you feel jittery, have headaches and contribute to high

blood pressure. Caffeine makes it more difficult to relax and fall asleep at night.
6. One must maintain a regular schedule of sleep even during very busy periods of life.
7. Smoking is bad for your health; it may cause you to feel more tired during the day. Nicotine is a stimulant; it increases the heart rate and blood pressure while causing insomnia. Like caffeine, nicotine may also cause your energy to crash and burn when the buzz goes away.
8. We are not always fortunate to have home-cooked foods. However, while eating out one should try to avoid fast food, oily and spicy food. Sweet dishes made from concentrated sugar should be avoided as much as possible.
9. I truly believe that the best way to keep your heart, mind, and soul healthy is by being with nature. A beautiful connection with nature brings joy, happiness and positive vibes. No matter how low you feel, nature has a way to turn things around.
10. Keep good connections with doctors and pharmacists in your vicinity.

Life has a habit of throwing surprises and we should be prepared. These are some of the basic practices that should be incorporated into one's regular lifestyle to avoid health complications. One should always follow the advice of doctors and abide by the various regimens of medications that they prescribe but it is also necessary to keep a very composed mind. Whether one is healthy or ailing, it is necessary to follow a balanced emotional pattern. By getting ruffled over petty issues we often harm ourselves.

I take the liberty to encourage people who are fighting some ailment in their lives because I have recovered from one of the scariest diseases. I believe that if you have a strong will to live, the Universe is bound to support

> As we start aging we realize that health is the greatest wealth that we possess and so, it is mandatory that we sustain a sound mind and robust body.

you. Life is a wonderful blessing and worth living each minute. So, if you ever have negative thoughts, please do stay away with them. The Universe and God support life and it is a privilege to live. If you believe in yourself, your grit to live your life will definitely be rewarded. If you look around with positivity in mind, you will feel the unconditional support that the world is offering you. Remember that half the battle is always won by the mind-be it a war or a deadly disease. If we believe that we can recover, ultimately, we will!

Today, my disease is something of the past. My once-upon-a-time shaven head is full of hair (hair re-grows within 4-6 months after the last cycle of chemotherapy) and my life is slowly coming back to normalcy. However, the disease has taught me some valuable life lessons and a world of knowledge.

I would like to tell you a story that many of you might have come across earlier. It is very appropriate for the topic I am discussing here. The 'Shocking Rat Experiment' teaches us powerful life lessons; it is basically a story of hope and belief.

In a series of experiments that were fairly cruel and unpleasant, Dr. Curt Richter of John Hopkins University demonstrated that hope is a powerful factor in perseverance. In our view, this is also closely linked with resilience. Ritcher's experiment focused on how long it would take for a rat to drown and die. He conducted his experiment by placing rats into buckets filled with water and seeing how long they survived. He introduced a range of variables into the experiment.

Experiment One: Richter put rats into big buckets, half-filled with water. Even being good swimmers—the rats on average give up and drown after 15 minutes.

Experiment Two: In experiment 2, he does something different. Just before the rats gave up due to exhaustion, the researcher would pull them out, dry them off, and let them rest for a few minutes. And then he would put them back into the water again for the second round. On this second try, how long do you think the rats lasted?

Another 5 minutes?

10 minutes?

15 minutes?

60 hours!

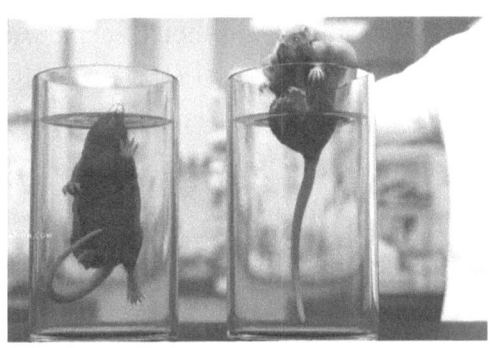

That's right! 60 hours of swimming. Because the rats believed that they would eventually be rescued, they used every ounce of energy in their body to push away death.

Hope is seeing light despite being surrounded by darkness. If hope can make frustrated rats swim for 60 hours long, what could belief in your abilities and yourself, do for you?

Humans and rats are very different beings but there is still a belief that we can learn a lot from these experiments. Those individuals who have hope have higher levels of perseverance. They will keep fighting until they find a chance of success or rescue. When they don't have hope, they won't fight and will easily give up which ultimately leads to fatality.

Such experiments in life teach us a valuable lesson about never giving up hope. It is the harbinger of life and your entire body system acts as per your command to be positive and hopeful or negative and hopeless. One has to always choose the former and never let hopelessness inflict unbearable pain. I am now more at peace with myself and I suggest that everyone practice a controlled lifestyle.

Today, we have a lot of technological interventions happening all over the world, but sometimes too much technology also disturbs our inner harmony. We should keep ourselves updated about the happenings around us. However, too much exposure to television or other media often lets negativity sneak into our lives. In this changing world order, we should be tech-savvy but not hinder our daily lives by becoming tech-slaves.

When used in excess, even the versatility of mobile phones or the internet is harmful. The mind yearns for relaxation after a hard day's toil. It is our responsibility to provide the necessary rest to our minds by having regular and proper sleep during the night and nourishing it with healthy food. As time passes and we start aging, we realize that health is the greatest wealth that we possess and so it is mandatory that we sustain a sound mind and a robust body.

Though one may never predict ailments, we should safeguard ourselves as much as we can. Neither my family members nor I had ever imagined that I could have cancer. However, even when I was diagnosed with cancer, I was able to maintain the discipline to get over it. So, despite leading a normal lifestyle, if you do get some health problems, do not despair or be depressed. There are bigger plans about to be revealed. I will reveal everything in the following chapters.

Points to ponder:

- Life is uncertain and therefore, one must live and cherish the present.
- Always remember good lessons and values from the past.
- Always spend quality time with family.
- Accept your circumstances and never remain in denial. Work out a solution and overcome the problem.
- Strong people are tested through tough times. If you are going through a tough period, remember that you are strong.
- Try spending more time with positive people.
- Believe that you can swim to the shore despite all adversities.
- Always have faith in God. He has greater plans for you.
- Block and delete all contact with negative people.

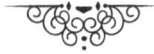

> Belief that you can swim to the shore despite all adversities will help in winning the race of life.

PHASE 2
THE DETECTION

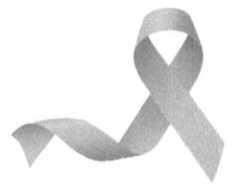

EARLY SYMPTOMS

"Life is under no obligation to give us what we expect." I feel that this particular line from Margaret Mitchell's book *Gone with the Wind* is appropriate and will set the tone for this chapter.

My beloved, visionary father who had been a great source of inspiration for all of us had left for his heavenly abode in August 2012. Ever since, we have all been meeting in Sonagiri, Delhi, Kolkata or Bengaluru to pay respectful tribute to him every year during August.

One day in August 2021, along with my wife and other family members, I was at my younger brother's home in Delhi. We have always been eager to attend every family gathering, ritual and festival together. A religious ritual was planned to pay our respectful tribute to our father. It was his 9th death-anniversary and this time we decided to gather in Delhi as my mother was also there at that time. It has become an annual ritual and we look forward to the occasion, though it is a solemn one.

Normally, it is an affair of a day or two and I had not planned for any prolonged stay, nor did I have plans of returning to Delhi soon but fate had other plans which I was unaware of.

EARLY SYMPTOMS

Soon after the rituals, while in Delhi, I felt some discomfort in my throat while swallowing. I tried to ignore it thinking it was a seasonal issue but when it persisted, I consulted my niece, Dr. Noopur, and son-in-law, Dr. Ankit Jain. They suggested I gargle with salt and warm water since it is the most common remedy for throat irritation. I followed their advice but could not rid myself of the problem and after returning to Kolkata, I observed a swelling in my throat that was perceptible and more visible. That day for the first time I was concerned about the irritation not being cured by the usually effective home remedies.

On 25th August 2021, I consulted my family physician, Dr. Bijay Patni. After a patient checkup and hearing, he recommended a round of antibiotics as the treatment since he too did not comprehend it to be a serious matter. I meticulously completed the course as per his advice but nothing seemed to improve. Though the lump in my throat was not causing much pain, its very presence brought a feeling of discomfort. I got annoyed by the persistent presence of the swelling every time I couldn't stop myself from reaching out to feel it.

I have never had any serious illness in my life. I had never been admitted to a hospital. Though I didn't contemplate much about either of the eventualities, sometimes I wondered whether the swelling would ultimately require surgery to be removed. I relegated all negative thoughts to the background whenever they emerged in my mind to cause worry. Even after completing the course of antibiotics, the problem remained and the recurrent thought was that it might not be a common irritation. I only hoped that it wasn't anything sinister.

I visited Dr. Patni again and he advised me to get an ultrasound done immediately to check the problem in more detail. Though he tried re-assure me that it seemed to be something that could be resolved through medicines. The ultrasound was done on the 3rd of September 2021.

The report was received in the evening of 4th September 2021 and it read as below:

Left lobe thyroid nodule (T1-RADS 5)
Discrete left parathyroid and left cervical nodes (level III, IV) with loss of central echogenic hilum.

The report suggested guided Fine Needle Aspiration Cytology (FNAC) from the left lobe thyroid nodule and left cervical node.

The medical terminologies were not familiar to me but the expression on Dr. Patni's face had changed drastically after seeing the report. He immediately advised me to get FNAC done with a tone laced with anxiety and concern. I have known Dr. Patni for the past 15 years and have always seen him to be calm and composed. Therefore, his worried demeanor and his anxiety made me uncomfortable. The same evening, I decided to get another opinion on it from Dr. Balram Prasad, who is a renowned general physician in Kolkata. Despite it being late at night, he came back to see me in his chamber. He was of the same opinion about getting FNAC done at the earliest.

The next day, I continued with my daily routine and went for a morning walk. I tried my best to treat the day as normal as I could because by getting anxious, I would only cause more panic in my family.

EARLY SYMPTOMS

After lots of contemplation and discussions amongst ourselves, we decided to fly to Delhi on the same day for further consultations with doctors there. I flew with my wife and reached Delhi at night. My younger brother, Sushil, and his wife, Sandhya, who were also very worried, came to receive us at the airport. I felt that it was important to get advice from someone close to us to calm our nerves. So, we went to Dr. Sanjay Jain who is an ENT expert at the Batra Hospital. He is my wife's cousin and I knew that his expert advice would be genuine and authentic. After giving a patient hearing and studying the earlier reports, he also suggested I get the FNAC test done at the earliest.

FNAC is a reasonably simple and quick method that is used for sampling perceptible growths and is usually performed in the Outpatient Department (OPD) with no requirement for hospitalization or surgery. It causes minimal pain and discomfort for the patient and generally does not create any complications. Growths located within the region of the head, neck as well as in the salivary gland and thyroid gland lesions can be readily diagnosed through this technique. The objective of this descriptive study was to determine the frequency of various pathological conditions detected through ultrasound which was otherwise not able to be observed.

It is concluded that tuberculosis lymphadenitis is still the commonest condition in patients presenting with neck swellings followed by non-specific lymphadenitis and malignant neoplasms and especially metastatic carcinoma. FNAC is, therefore, one of the easiest and most appropriate methods for the assessment of patients with neck swellings in the OPDs. Although its diagnostic accuracy cannot be compared to tissue biopsy, it is a good test for both screening and initial-level detection.

It is not prescribed for seemingly common cases and so my family got anxious over the diagnosis. I almost asked the doctor whether it was a tumor or something malignant. The curious part was that the swelling did not cause much pain. It was only an object of discomfort especially while swallowing food or saliva. So, confusion prevailed. I sometimes wondered why the doctors weren't proposing a microsurgery to remove the lump once and for all. However, I realized that the throat is a highly sensitive location to try out anything adventurous. With the presence of the windpipe and the esophagus, the throat is a vulnerable region of the body. A small mistake can result in huge damage.

I started craving sweets, which was an abnormality in my food habits. It wasn't that I was born with a sweet tooth but suddenly I had been having an intolerable urge to gorge on sweet dishes that are easily available in Kolkata. This temptation had a specific reason that I didn't know about then. Meanwhile, I decided to stay in Delhi to get the other required tests done. The decision was mainly based on the fact that in Delhi, I had my younger brother and his family along with numerous relatives and friends to make me feel at home. And above all, my caring mother was there. Though we had not revealed anything specific to her, her presence always kept my spirits very high. I wanted to be with my near and dear ones from them I could derive strength to combat an unknown malady.

After various rounds of discussions with different doctors, I was convinced that the process would not be a short-term stint and therefore, we decided to go to a place that would give us definite and assured results. One such center was Medanta-The Medicity Hospital in Gurgaon. It is the topmost and best specialty medical center in India. With world-class infrastructure, facilities, specialized doctors and nurses, it has grown in stature rapidly in the Indian medical field. As mentioned previously, my younger brother's son-in-law, Dr. Ankit Jain, was working in Medanta and his presence was a huge confidence booster. I had also read a few articles from authentic sources regarding this hospital right from its very inception and therefore, I had developed great conviction in their credibility.

THE INVESTIGATION

It is often said that rain helps us appreciate the rainbow. That's true for even human life. Regardless of how meticulously we plan our lives, trials come out of nowhere and cause painful situations. Dealing with uncomfortable situations is never easy. Facing problems and struggling to get back on track are simply inevitable. But no matter the struggle, you have the power to overcome anything through perseverance and strength. It's important to remember that nothing is permanent that this too shall pass, and that your resilience will grow.

On the 6th of September 2021, accompanied by my wife, Suman, brother, Sushil and his wife, Sandhya, I made our way to Medanta Hospital in Gurgaon through the chaos of traffic and emotions. It indeed took utmost patience to bear the heavy traffic, honking and rashness on the road while on a drive from Delhi to Gurgaon in rush hours. My eldest son, Harsh and daughter-in-law, Shilpa, had also arrived there for the meeting with Dr. Deepak Sarin, a specialist in head and neck oncology.

I had been leading a balanced and disciplined lifestyle from an early age. Going to a hospital for my health issues, and that too, in the oncology department was beyond my wildest dreams. Hence, this was a unique experience for me. The 10th floor of the hospital was dedicated to oncology with a large team of doctors, nurses and other caregivers present at all the places that could be perceived. The floor was also teeming with patients who were in various phases of treatment. The place was abuzz with activity that was in stark contrast to the activities that I had been accustomed to. It appeared to be a different world altogether.

When I stepped on to the floor, I was stunned to see so many patients in one hospital, that too, in a single floor. I saw small babies as well as the elderly suffering from cancer and at the mercy of fate and the doctors. From their faces, I could see that some were struggling to live while others were struggling to conclude their lives. The family members who had accompanied the patients had gloomy faces and pained expressions. We waited through the heavy haze of gloom to await our turn to be called by the doctor. It appeared to be a perennial wait as the long minutes of the watch ticked on.

Finally, our turn came to see Dr. Deepak Sarin and after a brief set of discussions, he examined the reports and after having a look at the swelling, he suggested an immediate FNAC.

I had been mentally ready for the test for some time and was soon led to OT. The pathologist appeared highly professional to me while laying out the procedures for the test. It might have been a mundane job for him but for a person undergoing the process for the first time, it is of paramount importance. Millions of thoughts stormed my mind as he readied his needle and handle to pierce through the lump to extract the required sample for further observation. Though the pathologist assured me of a pain-free procedure, I found his assurances quite hollow as the needle lanced through the skin almost making me squirm and yelp. The procedure ended much before I could reach the limits of my tolerance and I felt relieved even though the tingling pain persisted even after he informed me that the task was over.

Along with my family members, I proceeded to register for the CT scan; which was done much sooner than expected. After these procedures, I was informed that the reports would be available on the next day. So, we headed back to Delhi.

Our car managed to weave through the traffic as we dodged the vehicles on the road and the countless anxious questions that came up in my mind. I had nothing to say at home except for the strange experience and the process of the tests. Only a handful of people in my family knew why these tests were done. My grandchildren and mother were kept aloof from the looming reality.

The wait was excruciating. Just like any other night awaiting the result of an examination, this too was a long one. Weird thoughts kept running through my mind even after I tried hard to keep them at bay. I had decided back at the hospital that come what may, I would never lose my composure, cheerfulness or patience at any moment during the process of diagnosis and treatment. As I tried to get into the elusive slumber, I was further determined not to give up on my gritty resolve and unflinching faith in God's decisions. I kept promising myself earlier that I would never detach from positivity and hope, and would face the situation whatever the test results. Furthermore, I wanted to assure my close ones of positive results as I didn't want them to suffer emotionally because of me.

It was indeed a difficult night and I got to sleep quite late after anxious moments of tossing around in bed. However, I was awake

THE INVESTIGATION

quite early and was through with my morning chores much before the daily timings. I teamed up again with my wife, my son and my brother after breakfast and got ready to tolerate the torturous traffic en route to Medanta Medicity. On the way, I tried to exude cheerfulness and humor to lighten up the tense faces that were accompanying me. Sometimes, the ploy worked and sometimes it didn't.

We could collect the report after a short wait. The report spelled out the words, "**Suggestive for Lymph Proliferative Disorder.**" There was nothing specifically stated in the whole report, which made us further confused as we resorted to seeking more explanation from the doctor.

Dr. Deepak Sarin, however, did not seem much surprised by the report and was unable to douse our anxiety. We had hoped that the FNAC and scan would draw the necessary inferences for the swelling and that we would soon be able to follow the proper procedures for the treatment.

However, Dr. Sarin explained that the FNAC was not conclusive and that they were unable to arrive at any clear diagnosis. Therefore, a Tru-Cut biopsy was required for a final diagnosis. A Tru-Cut biopsy involved the use of a needle consisting of an outer cannula with a serrated rod on the inside. The surgeon would use the interior rod to cut the tissue specimen, trap it inside the cannula, and withdraw the entire needle containing the specimen for investigation.

I had no other option but to follow the instructions of the doctor to arrive at a conclusive result. Once again, we returned home, meandering through the traffic to wait for another set of tests to have a definite assessment. The anxiety at home had been increasing with each passing hour and everybody keenly waited and prayed for some positive result to emerge from the tests. My son, Harsh, had been vigorously searching the internet regarding the tests, procedures, various case studies and alternative sources to equip him more with the terminologies and processes. At times, I questioned how we could have combated such diseases without the help of advanced-level tests and the internet. The availability of information on the internet is nothing less than a boon. In the near future, with further developments in technology, the next generation will surely have more comfortable access to information and medical treatments.

Dinner that evening started on a quiet note. Everybody seemed to be lost in their thoughts and some of them seemed to be quite restless too. However, to lift the pall of gloom, I decided to talk about a few funny topics that I could remember. It did very little to lift the mood of the people.

The faces again regained their seriousness the next day as we neared the massive infrastructure of the hospital. I, too, braced myself for another grueling battle with pain to sustain the procedure of the Tru-Cut biopsy. I entered the same floor and the scene did not seem much more appalling this time. Had I got accustomed to such a vision or had I accepted myself to be within the same fraternity of helpless sufferers? I didn't delve into much soul-searching as we were soon ushered into a separate room for the test procedures.

The Tru-Cut biopsy was to be conducted with a much thicker needle to get more tissue samples for a clearer diagnosis. The needle itself looked ominous and I twitched a little to display my discomfort. The surgeon informed me that I would be anesthetized with local

THE INVESTIGATION

anesthesia before the actual process. It somewhat soothed me. Soon, the expert hands of the surgeon got busy in the process and he completed his task in a rather systematic manner. My throat was still numb when I got out of the surgeon's room. I inquired about the time required for the report to come but the doctor did not give any definite answer and indicated that they would try to get it as soon as possible.

We made frantic calls to the hospital every morning, afternoon and evening to know the status of the report and each time we were informed that it was on its way. It made us almost paranoid to hear the same reply repeatedly but we had no option but to wait for a more positive and definite reply. Due to the delay and prolonged wait, the pall of gloom had not lifted from my household.

Everybody seemed upset about the delay and as the days passed, the anxiety grew to ominous proportions. Although I was also quite disturbed during the waiting period, I knew that the onus was on me to keep the spirits of the household high. It is rather painful to see your near and dear suffer silently due to the concern they have for you and I was no exception to this. I tried to keep everybody jovial with lighthearted talk, cracking jokes, playing with each other, etc. People around me tried doing the same too. I could feel the extra politeness, concern and care in whatever they said or did to me. The entire family was together to fight this battle.

The much-awaited report finally arrived after six days on 13th September 2021. We had all expected the report to be in great detail and understood that time was being taken to bring out an elaborate and extensive report. It was shocking that even this report was inconclusive in giving a clear diagnosis.

The report read:

Left thyroid nodule: Scanty lesions tissue.

Overall features are suggestive of a Lympho-proliferative lesion likely Classical Hodgkin's Lymphoma.

Once again, the report did not soothe our nerves due to its inconclusiveness. Despite trying very hard to keep my mind calm, my family members and I were mentally disturbed. It felt as if I was circling around without any concrete solution.

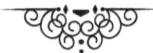

THE FINDINGS

I was confused by the mystery of the specialists' inability to recognize the magnitude of the problem. The seemingly innocuous swelling had taken even renowned practitioners in the field by surprise. It made me remember the vitality of the Corona Virus. Though it started out as just another virus, it had thrown the world into a tizzy in its effort to map its characteristics and its capacity to cause harm. Even my ailment seemed like a nameless nemesis. To gather more knowledge than the inadequate wording in the report I talked to several specialists on the subject. A proper and satisfactory understanding was still elusive.

After several rounds of discussion and brainstorming, the doctors came to the conclusion that an even larger biopsy sample was required to get a definitive diagnosis. We were advised to send our tissue samples to Dr. Anita Borges, a renowned cancer pathologist and a retired Professor, who has been in charge of surgical pathology at the famous Tata Memorial Hospital in Mumbai. She is a top histopathologist in India, who is based in Mumbai and is recognized as an authoritative figure in cancer pathology. She has handled many critical cases and seemed to be the right person to consult given the circumstances. Without much delay, we sent both the FNAC and the Tru-cut biopsy samples to her lab. While the reports were under process, I got my PET scan done on the 14th of September 2021. The scan discovered the presence of a mass in the left thyroid gland.

I met the Padma Shri awardee, Dr. Ashok K. Vaid, Chairman of the Medical Hematology Oncology Cancer Institute of Medanta, with the reports of the PET scan. He advised me to wait for the reports from Dr. Anita Borges. I realized that even core specialists wanted to be absolutely sure before coming to a conclusion.

Every doctor, nurse, caregiver and other related medical staff member has the huge responsibility of communicating the right message in the most appropriate way. I understood that doctors don't generalize the cases that require grave attention. Though they might have handled multiple cases in the past, they always treat each case as a new one. They knew that their verdicts might change the lives of the patients and their families. Therefore, they take the time and are cautious before announcing any result.

In fact, proper communication is of paramount importance in the case of health and illness. Humans are emotional beings. A wrong or misconstrued message may go a long way to wreck a family. Medical practitioners should also remember to give every patient the due attention. A patient who feels neglected or ignored, generally, goes into depression making the process of recovery all the more difficult. Fortunately, in my case, none of the doctors had given any wrong advice or diagnosis.

Reports from Dr. Anita Borges came on the 21st of September 2021. Her initial finding was completely different from the Medanta reports and she asked for a larger sample as well for a clearer

THE FINDINGS

diagnosis. She suggested that it was more likely to be an **EBV-related diffuse large "B" Cell Non-Hodgkin Lymphoma**, which would require an entirely different line of treatment. Our learning from this ordeal was that one should always take multiple expert opinions and not try to rush into treatment for the sake of running out of time. I also learned that even experts may misjudge and make mistakes while diagnosing and one should not jump to conclusions from a single source.

Whatever initial information we could collect was from the knowledge shared on the website of the Mayo Clinic, which reads like this:

Non-Hodgkin's lymphoma is a type of cancer that takes place in the lymphatic system, which is part of the body's immune system and fights all pathogens and germs. In non-Hodgkin's lymphoma, white blood cells called lymphocytes grow abnormally and in an uncontrolled way and can form growths, tumors or lumps throughout the body.

Non-Hodgkin's lymphoma is a general category of lymphoma. There are many subtypes that fall into this category. Diffuse large B-cell lymphoma and follicular lymphoma are among the most common subtypes. The other general category of lymphoma is Hodgkin's lymphoma which is very different in texture and can be easily detected. Advances in the diagnosis and treatment of non-Hodgkin's lymphoma have helped improve the prognosis for people with this disease.

It also described the symptoms as **'Swollen lymph nodes'** as the primary symptoms.

Signs and symptoms of non-Hodgkin's lymphoma may include:

- Swollen lymph nodes in the neck region, armpits or groin
- Abnormal pain in the Abdomen or swelling
- Chest pain, coughing or trouble breathing
- A persistent feeling of fatigue
- Frequent Fever
- Night sweats
- Unexplained weight loss

I learnt that these are two similar types and forms of cancer that are often confused. They are Hodgkin's Lymphoma and Non-Hodgkin's Lymphoma. Both of these forms of cancer affect the lymphatic system, which carries the fluid of the vital medium called lymphocytes. These lymphocytes contain white blood cells which fight infections and safeguard the immune system of the body.

The name of it has been derived from Dr. Thomas Hodgkin who detected cancerous lymph nodes way back in 1832. The disease attained the pseudonym 'Hodgkin's disease' until it was officially rechristened as 'Hodgkin's Lymphoma' in the late 20th century. Both forms of this cancer have similar symptoms, however, Hodgkin's Lymphoma is easier to treat because of the presence of Reed-Sternberg lymphocytes, which a physician can identify using a microscope. In Non-Hodgkin Lymphoma, these cells are absent and thus, the spread becomes unpredictable.

This unpredictability was the terrifying factor that made it difficult to ascertain the type that had taken shape. However, it is essential to learn that, nowadays, the survival rate for any type of cancer is much higher than a decade ago. So, it is advisable that in the case

THE FINDINGS

of any swelling or inflammation in the body that persists for longer than usual, one should immediately get it checked and have tests done on it. It might or might not be cancer, but there is no harm in getting it tested!

The inconclusive reports had sent the entire family into emotional turmoil. We felt like we were being made to go around in circles with no definite direction. One biopsy after the other with no conclusive result, it was making us feel helpless. There was little that could be done apart from following the instructions of the doctors and hoping for a definite answer. At that moment, my bigger challenge was to not let our disappointment turn into panic.

Soon, we scheduled a Tru-cut biopsy for a larger sample with Dr. Deepak Sarin. This time, my younger son, Abhinandan, was there to look after me and he supported the family and me throughout the process and its aftermath. The report of the biopsy came on the 30th of September 2021 and was much in line with what Dr. Anita Borges had suggested. It was finally confirmed that I had a rare type of cancer.

We went to meet Dr. Ashok Vaid the next day with the hope of starting the treatment as soon as possible as we had been informed that this is a very aggressive form of cancer. Even Dr. Ashok Vaid, in all humility and graciousness, suggested corroborating this report once again with Dr. Anita Borges, to confirm the correctness of the diagnosis.

We sent these samples to Dr. Borges and got the reports for them by the 7th of October 2021. The diagnosis was confirmed to be:

EBV associated non-Hodgkin lymphoma of large 'B' cell type (non-GC subtype by Hans' algorithm) with a double expresser phenotype (MYC+ Bcl 2+).

My entire family was shattered by the knowledge of such a disease since it was something that had happened for the first time in our family. Everyone was unsure about choosing the most appropriate place and hospital for the successful treatment of such a malignant problem. Though there were many contrasting revelations available on the internet, we wanted guidance from proper case studies to select the best of hospitals.

The atmosphere at home had a look of utter despondency and people prayed frantically to defeat the malignant malaise. I admit that I too had been shaken, but my pristine faith in God and strong self-belief allowed me to find the courage to face the problem head-on. The verdict had thrown my people into delirium, but somewhere from within I knew that this was a temporary problem and I would emerge from this situation soon. Since we now knew about the disease, we could approach a good specialist for the right treatment.

I have had to confront grave challenges many times in my career. My adventurous nature and courageous abilities in decision-making have helped me overcome most of the challenges. However, this was a different and more malicious challenge. Nevertheless, at no point in time did I feel overpowered by this adversary. I knew it could also be sorted out with time.

Under testing circumstances, our best friend is our own self-belief. Circumstances always tend to challenge our belief systems. However, if one is strong and determined, even strong gusts of

THE FINDINGS

wind are inadequate to extinguish the flame. Life is for living, not just staying in constant fear of the inevitable. We all know that we will die one day, but living in fear of death jeopardizes the boon of life that we are bestowed with.

COVID restrictions made commuting difficult but due to the ease of communicating through various online platforms, we could consult with doctors, especially cancer specialists, sitting far and wide. In fact, Harsh & Abhinandan connected with many specialists online to attain new ideas to arrest the scourge and had always kept me updated on their findings. I am really grateful to God, who has bestowed on me such a wonderful family. It is indeed a magnificent blessing to have loving and caring family members around you.

Though my long absence from the office caused some curiosity, my brother and my sons managed to keep the situation under control. Harsh and Abhinandan had been working strategically to create a strong system for the smooth functioning of our business. This was the time when their hard work was paying dividends. My absence never had any effect on our business. In fact, when many companies were struggling to cope with the backlash of COVID, our company was making steady progress. I kept myself updated about our business activities and could understand two very important things in the process.

1. To run a successful company, one must have a strong system in place. Systems and processes are very important to run a company seamlessly.
2. If proper SOPs are in place, no one is indispensable since the system itself manages the affairs of the company.

Initially, my family was not able to decide which hospital and city to start my treatment. I wanted my treatment to happen at a location where I could feel more comfortable. Delhi and Mumbai appeared to be possible places. However, before making a final choice we wanted to check out the facilities at the famous Tata Memorial Cancer Institute in Mumbai. Of course, there was no harm in checking but, within me I derided the idea of shifting to Mumbai. Though I had visited the city numerous times and had many friends and associates there, I was somehow unable to identify myself with the city. However, I was not willing to make my own choices. My family members were too anxious to get me to the best treatment. Therefore, I needed their concurrence to choose the right location and hospital to start my treatment.

Hope is a powerful force. It inspires us to do the impossible and helps us carry on during difficult times. And hope can come in many different forms. It may be through our favorite music, a good book, or even listening to our favorite thought leaders. One must never relinquish hope even during the most critical times. In fact, I realized that the divine is giving me a message to release my worries and stress and the divine will itself work out the best plan for my life.

I had no idea how the disease would be cured, what kind of treatment I would need to go through, or for how long. I had to summon all my mental and emotional resources to face the thoughts of the unknown that emerged in my mind. Would I succeed in doing so?

I was a little worried about the thought. But my mind reminded me of the lines, "And then I realized that to be more alive, I had to be less afraid." So, I did it. I lost my fear and regained my whole life.

> "The human spirit is stronger than anything that can happen to it."
>
> C.C. Scott

THE BEGINNING OF TREATMENT

My sons, Harsh and Abhinandan, had rushed to Mumbai along with Shailesh Jain, our family friend, who had faced a similar stressful experience with his mother's ailment. They had consulted several doctors and were trying to find the best doctor for my treatment. They met Dr. Manju Sengar at Tata Memorial Hospital, who is an onco-hematology specialist in lymphoma and decided that her expert treatment would be the most appropriate for me. After that weekend, my entire family flew to Mumbai to support me while I embarked upon the journey of treatment to recovery.

In Mumbai, Mr. Ashok Patni, Chairman of RK Marbles & Wonder Cement, who is my nephew, Deepak's father-in-law, offered his wonderful flat in Samudra Mahal for our stay. Although the flat was spacious and had all modern facilities, the feeling of discomfort was recurrent in me. Staying in Mumbai would mean staying away from my mother and family and the journey for the next 4-5 months would surely be in isolation and that would be very difficult without emotional and psychological support. Since I did not have any close relatives in Mumbai except my nieces, the realization dawned upon me to take a quick and tough decision to move to

THE BEGINNING OF TREATMENT

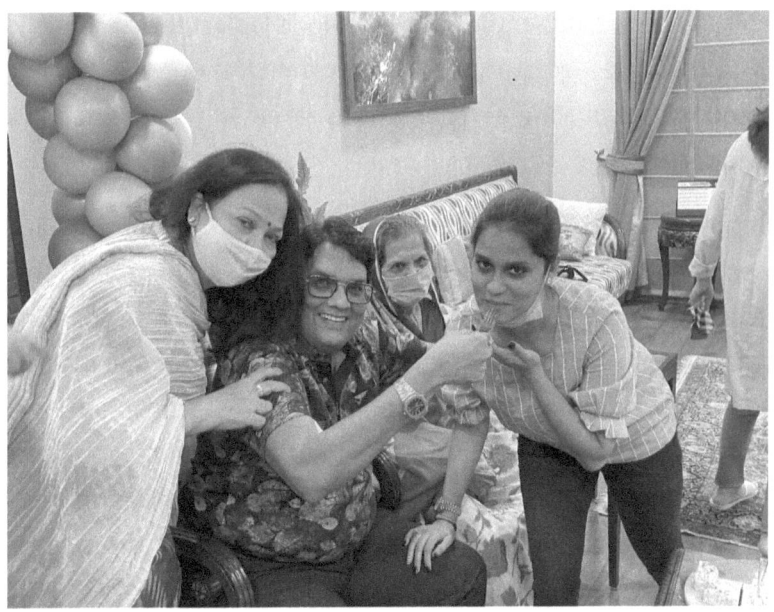

Delhi to be with my brother, his family and my mother during the course of the treatment.

Harsh had done all the initial discussions, preparations and had fixed my appointment with the doctor. I thought it would be hard and rigid on my part if I tell him that I would prefer treatment in Delhi rather than Mumbai as he worked relentlessly to find the best doctor, hospital, etc.

The next day, as per my appointment, we went to this specialty hospital in Mumbai. As soon as I reached the doctor's chamber, I felt uncomfortable being treated as an object. The doctor was more interested in looking into the various reports and the computer screens rather than conversing with the patient and family members. He seemed more engrossed with the plethora of case papers that were lying on the table and the screens of the computers, rather than having a good look at the patient and providing the necessary encouragement. Without even paying heed to the spiraling emotions, I was asked to get admitted in a nonchalant tone.

It seemed like I was in a robotic world, devoid of emotions and sentiments where the patients were merely treated as objects that had to undergo a process and come out alive or dead. The blinking computer screens and papers held more meaning to the modern world than proper humane communication systems. I was not convinced to be a part of this system of automation concerning human lives. And it was not only me, but the others who had accompanied me looked equally disagreeable to the system of robotic therapeutics.

I admit that the medical profession is a busy and overwhelming line among contemporaries. However, the importance of this profession brings with it huge responsibilities. It is important for a doctor or a caregiver to adequately communicate with the patients and their families to make them feel confident and comfortable with the system they are about to follow. Human emotion is a fact that should never be neglected. In fact, the humane behavior of a doctor or a caregiver goes a long way towards patients wellness. The message should be loud and clear, "Yes, we care for you and it is our prime responsibility to help you recover."

In the evening, we had a round of discussion regarding the various possibilities for the treatment. Though I didn't voice my opinion much, it was unanimously decided that my treatment would be done in Delhi where I would also get the love and care of my mother, brother and his family. This would ensure a homely experience for me. Hence, the family flew back to Delhi the next morning, 13th Oct 2021, and we headed straight to Medanta from the airport, met with Dr. Ashok Vaid and began the formalities required to start the treatment.

Admitted at Medanta

As soon as I got admitted to the oncocare department of Medanta Hospital, as general precursors for treatment nowadays, all mandatory check-ups were done. It was during COVID and the pandemic was creating havoc. As per COVID protocol, special check-ups were also conducted. Before starting the treatment, it was mandatory to check if cancer cells were present in the bone marrow, for which a bone marrow biopsy was to be done on admission. Local anesthesia was applied to the skin. The doctor taking the sample explained to me that the bone would not be numb with this and to expect some pricking pain upon the insertion of the needle. A thick needle was pierced into my backbone to take the required tissue sample. Though I was told about a pricking pain, it was more of a stabbing experience but with the alertness of the doctor, albeit benign, I was prepared for it.

Once you are prepared for the pain, you do not feel the intensity of pain when the needle is inserted. The pain is all the more painful when it is all of a sudden and without warning. Fear of pain is sometimes worse than the pain itself.

I was supposed to undergo chemotherapy since that was the only prescribed treatment for my ailment. I had been prescribed six doses of chemotherapy with a gap of three weeks between each session for the body to endure the same. It is a long-drawn process where the regular veins cannot tolerate the toxicity of the chemical concoction that was going to be injected into my body. Hence, to enable this process, they had to insert a thin tube into my veins through which the medicines would directly reach the bigger arteries in the chest and then get pumped throughout the body. To obtain a successful result in the process of treating any type of cancer takes a concoction of the right chemicals in precise proportions. A little oversight might be catastrophic.

To insert the Peripherally Inserted Central Catheter (PICC) line, I had to go to the operation theatre to get it done under guided ultrasound. This PICC line was meant to be kept for the next few months until my last chemotherapy session.

When the thin tube was being inserted into my veins, I was deeply perturbed by the casual approach of the technicians who had been entrusted with the job. They were engaged in friendly chatter amongst themselves as the tube was being inserted. As I lay in anxiety over the next course of action, their trivial chit-chat greatly annoyed me. I observed the disturbing nonchalance these caregivers exhibit in front of their patients. I didn't intervene during the process since I didn't want to disturb their rhythm, but after the process, I couldn't refrain from telling the technicians that they should not engage in idle chatter and pay more attention to the task lest they make any errors. They informed me that it was their mundane duty and so, I did not need to worry about any mistakes being committed. I wondered why they made the patient sign a long list of conditions if they were so confident about their procedures.

THE BEGINNING OF TREATMENT

Though this might be an everyday affair for them, it is a personal and emotional experience for their patients. Every act from here hinges on life and death. Therefore, the gravity of such situations needs to be honored. It should be an important curriculum for the medical practitioners to ensure that their behavior complements the situation and that the patient's perspective is always given due importance.

Chemotherapy

I was prescribed the R-CHOP chemotherapy drugs, which were meant to be given in cycles that were 21 days apart. R-CHOP is the acronym for the combination of drugs that are used in chemotherapy for certain types of cancer mainly Non-Hodgkin Lymphoma. In R-CHOP, there are 5 chemicals, namely Rituximab (Rituxan), Cyclophosphamide, Doxorubicin Hydrochloride, Vincristine (Oncovin), and Prednisone. Out of these drugs, Doxorubicin is meant to be the most powerful chemotherapy drug ever invented. It is used to treat a whole variety of cancers as it kills cancer cells at every stage of their life cycle.

That very day I was administered a few concoctions of the five chemicals and the rest was to be given the next day. It was given through an IV very slowly in order to check my body's reaction to the drugs. They were monitoring my blood pressure and heart rate very closely.

Throughout this period when the drugs were injected, I was garnering the mental strength to accept the outcome—good or bad—and I left it to the wisdom of God. I believed that whatever He does, it is for some reason and this gave me the internal strength to accept the outcome of these chemicals that were being injected into my body. Of course, my entire family was beside me to give me the much-required moral and mental support that was necessary of that hour.

Before starting to inject the chemicals, it is mandatory to have an intramuscular injection (ITMT) in the body. This is generally injected at the back of the patient and into the bone. The injected fluids form a layer and prevent the chemo from reaching the brain. The procedure should be done by a trained surgeon/technician since it is necessary to drive the injection to the right place. Though the technician had informed me that he had applied local anesthesia as I had mentioned earlier, anesthesia has no effect on the bones. Therefore, the injection brings about a lot of pain. I had requested that the person to inform me before administering the injection so that I could mentally prepare myself to endure the pain.

> Though the chemo did not feel as fiery as it was presumed to be, I could feel the pangs of raging fire rushing through my veins. The defense reinforcers had been unleashed to exterminate the intruders. I had mixed feelings and wondered about the side effects of this concoction of chemicals rushing through my body.

THE BEGINNING OF TREATMENT

I felt a little heavy and somewhat uncomfortable. I had already been told about feelings of nausea, headache and insomnia that would play their roles during the process and the aftermath. However, apart from a light uneasiness from the internal warm sensation, I did not have to endure any grave side effects. During chemotherapy, a patient can have a lot of side effects. Therefore, at regular intervals, the patient is asked about any discomforts. Generally, cardiologists, neurologists and urologists are summoned if any irregularities are noticed in the pulse, heartbeat, nausea or urinary problems.

In the morning, Dr. Ashok Vaid came to my room and asked how I was reacting to the drugs. He was happy to see that I did not have any serious reactions to the medication. He checked me, saw my records and advised us to administer the most potent drug Doxorubicin immediately. This drug was administered very slowly over the course of 3-4 hours. After the completion of the dosage, I was asked to rest until evening to see if I had any side effects.

My wife had been chanting her religious mantras and was praying to God in all her earnestness. In the room, she also ensured that the *Bhaktambar Strotra*, one of the most powerful Jain mantras, was playing throughout the period. Definitely, spiritual powers were also working to get everything in order.

A psychiatrist also visited to make me mentally prepared for the aftereffects of chemo. After my first chemotherapy, I was discharged in the evening. I went to my home in Delhi to meet my loving family who were all eagerly waiting. It was a huge relief to have taken such heavy chemicals without much discomfort.

On receiving such powerful drugs which impact the blood counts of the patients severely, one is advised to always take the utmost care of their health since immunity is at its lowest during this time. With COVID creating havoc all around, my family took extra precautions to ensure I had a safe stay. I was not allowed to meet visitors and stayed in my room throughout all my activities. The doctors had advised us that chemotherapy could lead to various side effects that vary from patient to patient. These side effects could be anything like nausea, mouth ulcers, constipation or diarrhea.

> The doctors had advised us that chemotherapy could lead to various side effects which vary from patient to patient.

Complete rest was advised as weakness was an expected outcome. To enable a better recovery, the patient should be under no mental stress. I slept well since my medication contained heavy sedative components. For the next 6-7 days, I was low on energy. I also had restricted bowel movements which made me very uneasy. My mouth felt like it was losing its sense of taste which made eating my meals very unpleasant. A follow-up blood test after a week of chemo, as advised by the doctor, showed that my blood counts had been impacted. It was better than what the doctor had expected and he explained that this would get better before the next cycle of chemo.

THE BEGINNING OF TREATMENT

I noticed that during the successive cycles of chemo, I had been steadily losing my hair. Every morning, seeing my pillow littered with hair had become a common occurrence. In order to get rid of this distasteful sight every morning, one day, I decided to shave my head bald. This un-consulted, impulsive activity proved to be disastrous because it resulted in an allergic infection on my scalp. I had to rush to a dermatologist for the itchy rashes and with the medicine prescribed to me, I got relief.

The concoction of chemicals given in chemotherapy makes the body weak and vulnerable to infections. A little negligence may invite a bunch of infections into the body. Therefore, it is of utmost importance to stay safe, secluded and upbeat throughout the period. During the breaks between the succeeding sessions of chemo, I maintained a strict and healthy diet devoid of sugar, wheat or gluten and milk products and was confined to selective fruits and easily digestible diets.

I followed the diet plan advised by Mr. Luke Coutinho, a holistic and wellness coach and one of the best nutritionists in India. Mr. Coutinho has co-authored 2 books—"The Magic Weight Loss Pill" and "The Great Indian Diet." My family consulted him and after understanding my ailment and the requirements of my body, he and his team member, Ms. Ekta Vadagama, Senior Nutritionist and Healthcare Coach prescribed the following routine and diet:

Time	Food Plan
7:00 AM	10 minutes of Pranayam, Anulom Vilom Oil Pulling before brushing
7:30 AM	1 glass warm water with one tsp. of Moringa powder
After 15-20 minutes	Soaked nuts & dry fruits-2 walnuts whole, 3 almonds, 2 black dates/prunes
Breakfast 9 AM	1 cup of almond milk with 1 tbsp of homemade protein powder in it-daily
10 mins. Post B/F	2 soaked bitter apricot kernels
10 min. before lunch	Amla, turmeric & ginger shot
Lunch	2 khapli wheat paratha stuffed with grated onions, carrot, cabbage, sattu powder, and spices with 1 bowl of boiled moong sabji
10 min. post lunch	2 soaked bitter apricot kernels

After 45 min. of Lunch	1 glass of lemon water. Chew 1tsp ajwain-jeera-saunf (AJS) & drink lemon water after chewing
5:00 PM	1 cup soursop Tea + 1 bowl fruit (100-150 gms) with 1 tsp of raw unsoaked flax seeds & 1 soaked macadamia nut 1 cup herbed & roasted makhana or roasted poha chivda
8:00 PM	2 moongdal chilla-add grated veggies to it + 2 tbsp of avocado dip

I was feeling quite comfortable with this diet chart and I would highly recommend consulting an expert nutritionist if someone is diagnosed with such a terminal disease. Furthermore, one should follow their diet religiously. In fact, Mr. Luke Coutinho's team was in constant touch with me and whenever I was having any discomfort, they changed the diet plan and suggested other food intakes.

I also read and listened to motivating pieces of information and stayed away from sources of negative influences. However, the wait for the next session appeared to be a bit long. I was conditioning my mind to be strong enough to endure the treatment but it was also necessary for the body to adapt to new conditions. My family members at home had been putting in extra effort to look after my wellbeing, especially Suman who had turned into a strong mother figure. I felt like a child entrusted to her care. I couldn't help but admire how she went into detail about all the precautionary measures while attending to me.

During the second chemo session, I was more prepared to face the perils that I had escaped during the first session. As the drops slowly entered my veins, the same warmth gushed through my body. The sudden rush of chemicals can make any mortal twitch. However, the mental strength that I had developed over the years always came to my rescue to assure me of better results. After the chemo, I found my body weakening further. I wobbled while walking and at times, I would feel that my feet would give away. The doctor had assured me that the weakness would slowly go away in the next few days with proper rest and cure.

I realized that during the initial 7 days of chemotherapy, the body experiences a weakening effect. To monitor the impact on blood cells, the doctor recommended conducting several blood tests after this period to ensure the chemotherapy drugs are not harming the blood cells. The following 14 days are dedicated to the body's recovery, preparing it for the next cycle of chemotherapy.

I had been told that cancer cells feed on sugar and gluten. These cells usually grow quickly, multiply at a faster rate and require lots of energy. This also means that they need lots of glucose to support themselves. Glucose is the basic fuel that powers every single cell in our body. If we eat or drink things that are high in glucose, such as sweets and fizzy drinks, the glucose in them gets absorbed straight into our blood ready for our cells to use.

Although, it is not scientifically proven that a sugar-free diet lowers the risk of getting cancer or boosts the chances of survival if diagnosed. But it is advisable to cut down on sugar and gluten intake and add foods that are good sources of fiber and vitamins. No wonder I had been having a huge craving for sweets before I went for the checkup for the swelling in the initial days.

Cancer patients need to have a proper and balanced diet because the treatment can result in weight loss and put the body under a lot of stress. So, poor nutrition could hamper recovery or even be life-threatening. A balanced diet, proper rest and reading inspiring stories helped to improve my strength. I was ready with high spirits for the third round of chemotherapy.

After the third chemo, I started limping. I had my people to support me but even getting into a waiting car was a huge struggle. My family was concerned but the doctor assured us that this was a common condition after the third dose and that, once again, with proper rest, the body will recover soon. This time too he also warned us that the body's immunity shield was down. So, seclusion and a proper diet had to be strictly followed.

We knew and understood that we had to follow these instructions strictly. However, it felt as though we were being too harsh by not allowing any meetups with some well-wishers who had come from long distances to see me and wish me a quick recovery.

I realized during the chemo sessions that the body becomes exceedingly vulnerable because of the extraneous doses. The periods of rest and intense care that I received from my family had gotten my body back to a state where I was ready to take the successive doses on time. I wanted to complete the 6th and last dose of chemotherapy on time.

Meanwhile, the restrictions on COVID had become stricter. Delhi and other major cities were badly impacted. All health centers and hospitals, including Medanta, were flooded with COVID patients. The talk around was to improve people's immunity since the virus had been infecting people with low immune systems. With my immunity at an all-time low, it was probable that my chemo might get delayed due to the circumstances. I prayed that this did not happen since I did not want to prolong my treatment. I had stayed in Delhi so that I could redeem the strength of my body without unnecessarily exposing it.

I saw people traveling back to their homes via flight or train between successive chemotherapy sessions. I believed that it was a grave mistake that these people were committing. When the resistance of the body is low and susceptible to extraneous attacks from viruses, pathogens, etc., one must stay cocooned in a safe place to allow the body to get adequate rest and recuperation and also provide it with the necessary security. One must also remain stress-free during the chemo regimens.

It is natural to be worried about the uncertainties the future hold and the imminent side effects that will follow. However, thinking about the positive aspects of life and being thankful to God for keeping us alive is a certain way to retain the tranquility of the mind. I believe that this is a stage when one should learn to appreciate the things they might have missed during the rat race of working and attending to family affairs. I started feeling the blessings of life from my secluded disposition very frequently. The loving and caring family I had was something I couldn't thank God enough for. I am sure everybody needs to be loved and cared for and it is paramount to feel blessed when you have such people all around you.

Nature has a unique essence of care. Whenever our eyes meet natural greenery—the wonderful flowers, the playful birds and animals—our mind is automatically transported to a world of peace and tranquility. Life in solitude allows one to admire the qualities of a good human being. One learns to appreciate more, forgive more and love more.

I am a great believer in spirituality. Therefore, I enjoyed a lot of discourse on the subject by various spiritual leaders to further enhance my knowledge on the subject. Additionally, reading books has always been my favourite hobby. This was the time when I read many meaningful books which further added to the value system that I had always carried. Suddenly, I felt the silence murmur words of wisdom in my ears. I loved the smell of dawn and the caress of the morning breeze, the tiptoeing dusk after the sun had set in all its glory and I got enthralled by the lullabies of the moonlit nights. It appeared that life had presented me with all its color and magnificence to enjoy and be thankful for. These are the little things we continuously miss under the pretext of a busy life and remain ignorant about the wonder that nature provides.

> My fourth and fifth chemo was administered as per schedule and the experience was similar to the earlier sessions.

I was relieved when the doctor announced that the 6th chemo session would happen on the scheduled date. When I arrived for the chemo session in Medanta, the treating doctor and nurses were full of admiration. Though I could only smile back in reply, I realized that I had managed to undergo the treatment with incredible courage. This was probably something that the doctors too might not have expected.

The minutes ticked by as the drips of the chemical concoction streamed through my veins. The process no longer induces pain or fear. The faces of the people out there had become all too familiar to me by then. They had also been quite friendly with me. Every now and then, cutting across professional lines, the doctors, technicians and nurses would talk to me about our families, children and various other aspects of life.

They liked my penchant for having ready answers to some of the questions that intrigued them. I feel this is because I was well-read and adventurous with the experience of having travelled wide and far. In fact, my spirit of adventure induced me to take risks and stay calm during tumultuous periods. My keen interest in adventure had taken me to various places that had provided me with a variety of experiences. From the icicles of Harbin in China and Alaska in the U.S.A. to the snow-covered Antarctica, my adventurous spirit had taken me everywhere. However, through every unfamiliar circumstance in life, I remained calm and composed.

I recall a particular experience while on a flight that involved experiencing big air turbulence and shaking violently. Many passengers shrieked and trembled with fear. Even my wife held onto my hand with a strong grip while reciting all the mantras that she could recall. On the other hand, I kept my calm to push through that terrible experience. My only mantra was that destiny would decide each person's fate. Why fret about things that are not in our control and why not enjoy every moment as a new experience? These are the memories that somehow made me strong. It had sometimes occurred to me that God had chosen me to go through this experience and learn from it. I strongly believe that if things are under control then why worry? And if things are not in your control, even then why worry?

The end of the sixth session of chemo brought mixed feelings. Though I felt weak and vulnerable, I was relieved that I had been able to go through the entire process without much struggle. There was also a feeling of sadness that I would be missing the team that had been so dutifully, diligently and passionately attending to me during my chemo sessions. Through these periods of time, I developed an emotional bond with everyone. In turn, they too became fond of me and wished for my complete recovery.

Though the process of chemotherapy had ended, another important phase of getting my body accustomed to the new composition of chemicals and medicines had begun. This is a very important stage for a patient. Giving the body required time for recovery enables it to regain the strength and vitality it once possessed.

During my days of recovery, nature had been one of my most cherished partners. I felt the strength of nature's beauty as it refreshed and reinvigorated me to face the future. The blessings are innumerable and the same reminds us time and again that we have to conserve nature for ourselves and our future generations. There is a lot of talk about deforestation, the depleting ozone layer and the melting of the icebergs in the Arctic and Antarctica. However, instead of just forwarding alarming messages in WhatsApp, we have a responsibility to impart the lessons learned from nature and the great virtue of the same to our progeny in our own little way.

If I were to look at the positive side, another opportunity that arose was the chance to remain with the best company. This was my own self—the most important person in my life. Sitting alone and taking the time to be still and look within was a once in a lifetime experience that I had not previously experienced in my life.

There are a few things that I feel are important to share.

The Leading Causes of Fatal Illnesses:

Nowadays, a wide variety of fruits and vegetables are being cultivated with the frequent usage of harmful chemicals and artificial fertilizers which not only poison the produce but also destroy the natural mineral capacity of the soil. Sadguru Jaggi

THE BEGINNING OF TREATMENT

Vasudev Ji spread this powerful message about "Save the Soil" and created awareness amongst people across multiple nations by doing a solo motorcycle journey across 27 countries.

Manmade preservatives, flavours, colors and other toxic chemicals have been destroying the natural nutritional values of our food while simultaneously pushing the toxic ingredients into our bodies. This creates havoc inside our body by causing conflict with its natural systems.

Dramatic changes in food, products and the environment have created a society of nutritionally deficient and chemically toxic human beings. Truly speaking, all the food items that are available to us for consumption are drastically different and menial in comparison to the foods our ancestors used to enjoy during their time.

With the experience and learning I gathered during my treatment, I would suggest avoiding consumption of any form of direct sugar, white flour, processed oil, milk products and packaged food items as much as possible. This is the best option if we want to safeguard our health and well-being.

It is also advisable to check the composition of any packaged food or drink that might have unhealthy levels of sugar, fat or other chemicals. Fresh and seasonal fruits and vegetables should be preferred over packaged food. Apparently, sugar is the super-food for cancer cells. Hence, sweets and concentrated sugar should be taken in moderation.

Dr. O. Carl Simonton, a radiation oncologist, popularized the mind-body connection in fighting cancer, in his book *Getting Well Again*, first published in 1978. This book talks about some important aspects of cancer. The author has mentioned how visual imagery with positive mental images has had a beneficial effect on patients with advanced cancer. Keep your images and suggestions as positive, simple, clear and concise as possible. Then, repeat them as often as possible. Allow the subconscious to accept them as a command and implement them.

Feelings of anger, apathy, gloom and resentment weaken the immune system and cause damage to health. Positive thoughts of love, compassion, joy, and humour support good physical health and the wellness of the mind. It takes some effort and discipline, especially during tough times, to keep an open and positive mindset. However, the health benefits definitely make it worthwhile.

Strong social support including family relations, friendships, relations with health practitioners, romantic relationships and relations with spiritual leaders and figures are critical components of healthcare.

I regularly listen to the positive affirmations on *Health and Healing* by Bob Baker on YouTube and I strongly recommend that everyone devotes some time to listening to them every day.

Positive Affirmations for Health & Healing

I am healthy.

I am perfect, whole & complete.

I choose to be healthy.

THE BEGINNING OF TREATMENT

I choose to be vibrant.

I choose to be whole.

Every cell in my body vibrates with life-giving energy.

My mind is sharp.

My body is in perfect working order.

I am healthy in mind, body & spirit.

I am grateful for the healing that's happening right now.

I call forth perfect health.

I command healing energy to flow through me.

I let go of what doesn't serve me.

I give myself permission to heal.

I am healing inside and out.

I am patient with myself every day.

My body heals in its own time.

My body heals in divine order.

I am radiant, beautiful and strong.

I believe in my ability to heal.

My body is a temple of health and healing.

My body is a magnet for wholeness.

Now is the time to be healthy.

My body is in perfect alignment.

The cells of my body tingle with positivity.

I command my body to be healthy.

I listen to my body.

My body tells me what it needs.

My body is an intelligent energy system.

My body is a health-making machine.

My body is in harmony with itself.

My body knows how to support itself.

My body is attuned to the wisdom of the universe.

My body is in harmony with the universe.

I am perfect, whole, and complete.

Additionally, Dr. Norman Cousins, in his highly acclaimed bestselling book, *Anatomy of an Illness*, attributed his recovery largely to the positive manner in which he viewed his situation.

> Mind has great power to change the body physically. We have at our disposal the means to assist our body in healing and upgrading our health by giving suggestions to our body such as 'I am getting healthier and stronger.'

THE BEGINNING OF TREATMENT

You may be surprised about why I am referring to all these books which are already available on public platforms. I have been reading them even before my cancer diagnosis. But during the days when I was going through my chemotherapies, I devoted my quality time to reading and listening not only to inspirational books and stories, but I also did a fair amount of research on cancer and read the books written by different survivors and doctors. This was to gain knowledge and experience in handling the condition in a well informed manner. I am referring here to those books that I have read and benefited from.

While I was reading the book *Peace, Love and Healing* by Dr. Bernie Siegel, a retired surgeon, who writes and teaches about mind-body-medicine and the relationship between the patient and healing has written a beautiful message. A sense of purpose can do wonders for your health. Exceptional patients don't leave any emptiness. They leave examples of their own lives and the love they have inspired in those around them. A purpose helps you determine your values, set goals and tackle challenges. All these can benefit your health immensely.

One should always focus on transforming from being tormented by unspoken and unacknowledged emotions to having healthy and consciously chosen emotions.

I was unaware of my true self and this was a period when I realised the immense internal strength in me that helped me face this demon.

The time I spent with myself has made me realise to take life easy and create new beginnings.

A meaningful American proverb I wish to quote here greatly communicates our responsibility towards our future.

"We don't inherit the earth from our ancestors; we borrow it from our children."

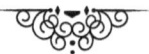

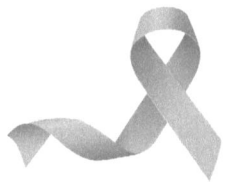

PILLARS OF STRENGTH

"One's family is the most important thing in life. I look at it this way: one of these days, I'll be over in a hospital somewhere with four walls around me. And the only people who'll be with me will be my family."- Robert Byrd

My long absence from Kolkata had triggered anxiety among the few who had always been accustomed to my company.

My grandchildren always treated me as a friend. Yuvan, Sanaya and Riaan had always been my best companions and had the habit of sharing everything with me. I was told that my little grandson, Riaan, who was just 3 years old, used to come searching for his *Dadu* and *Maa* (his grandmother) in our room several times every day without asking anybody at home. It was his tender love that prompted him to look for us during our absence.

In fact, I derived a lot of strength from each one of my grandchildren. My time in the company of my grandchildren was smooth and enormously enriching as they helped me cope with the pain effortlessly. The smiles, laughter and close bond that we shared amongst us were much more powerful than the pain I had to endure. I cannot thank God enough for providing me with such adorable grandkids.

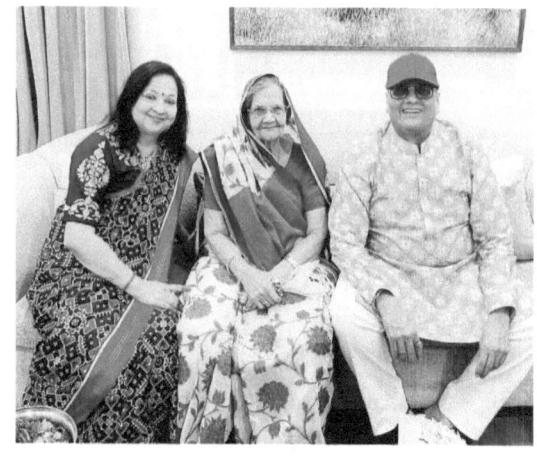

Like my late father, my mother is also exceptionally inspirational. My mother, who is 90 years old, is a very religious and spiritual lady. She is very particular about her routines and has the habit of having her meals before sunset. She doesn't eat or drink anything after 6 pm till 9 am the next morning. This has been her daily ritual for years and this practice, indeed, is very beneficial for her health. She is very caring and is concerned about everyone, young or old. Her deep belief in God has always inspired us to derive strength from the ultimate guardian who has unique ways to bring about the best results. She still uses her old sewing machine to stitch baby frocks and other useful items and she also knits socks and sweaters for the winter with much pleasure.

My wife, Suman Sethi, is a versatile homemaker. She has always taken a leading role in the house and has very passionately taken care of me during the entire duration of my treatment. She did not leave me even for a minute and was very particular about my medicines, timely meals, supplements and well-being. For the past 42 years, she has always been a great support for me but her exceptional support and care in the entire phase of my cancer investigation and treatment is highly appreciated.

It was her ardent mental, physical and emotional support that gave me the strength to face the after-effects of chemotherapies. I am known to be a problem solver in business circles and am sometimes eagerly sought after to provide solutions to tricky propositions. But I always look up to my mother and wife because I believe that they are better problem solvers than me. They have always come up with the most congenial solutions even in the trickiest of situations. During the most testing times of my life, she has proven why I consider her my better half.

My sons, Harsh and Abhinandan, were always there for me along with their wives, Shilpa and Priyanshi, during the entire treatment.

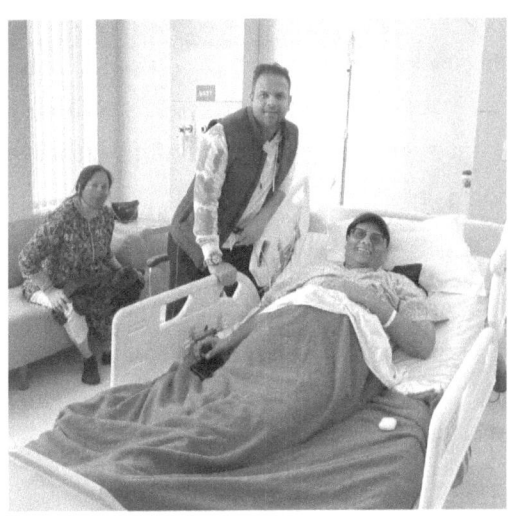

Despite having tight business schedules and professional commitments, Harsh handled all communication with the specialists in India and abroad and my treating doctors, nurses and technicians. My younger son, Abhinandan, was there with me in the hospital and took care of my treatment schedule. They are the support system that I can always count on.

My daughter, Roshni, and her daughter, Anaaita always travelled from their home in Bengaluru to Delhi whenever I had to go for my chemotherapies. She gave me great emotional support which is more than I expected from a lovable daughter.

My elder brother, Anil Sethi, his wife, Preeti Bhabi, my nephews, Deepak and Vineeta, my nieces, Jyoti and Pratibha and their husbands, Vikas Kothari and Sunny Pandya are very close to us even though they live in Bangalore and Mumbai. My brother had been particularly anxious throughout the treatment and when he was unable to come to Delhi, he made numerous calls to my younger brother, Sushil, and my sons to get an update about my recovery. He is also a very principled person and I have seen some glimpses of my father in his personality, time and again.

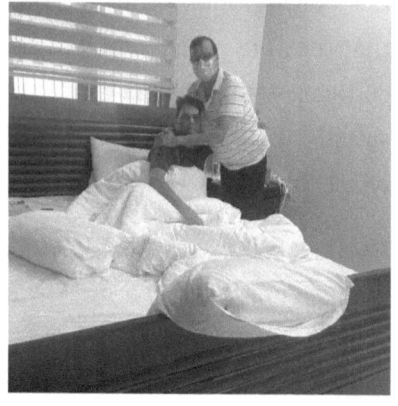

We have heard the saying, "Blood is thicker than water," which refers to how family relationships are stronger than the commitment you have to your friends and colleagues. I realized the true meaning of this when I landed in Delhi for my check-ups after the initial tests were done in Kolkata. My younger brother, Sushil and his wife Sandhya had taken care of me in such a way that Sushil often missed going to the office and important business meetings just to be with me. He literally shadowed me everywhere—from his home to doctors' clinics to hospitals.

I do not remember spending so much time with him after our childhood as we have both been busy with our work and making plans and strategies to take our company to greater heights. Ourconversations over the telephone for the past few years were mostly limited to our work, new projects, bank commitments and all topics centred on water—the sector we are catering to through our company. But when the time came to test the depth of the two brothers' love and affection for each other, he proved it beyond limits. There is a smile on my face when I am writing this as things have changed now. We both speak daily or several times a day and during all our conversations, we discuss everything under the sun except official matters. Both of us have handed over all work-related responsibilities to our sons and they are handling business affairs more diligently.

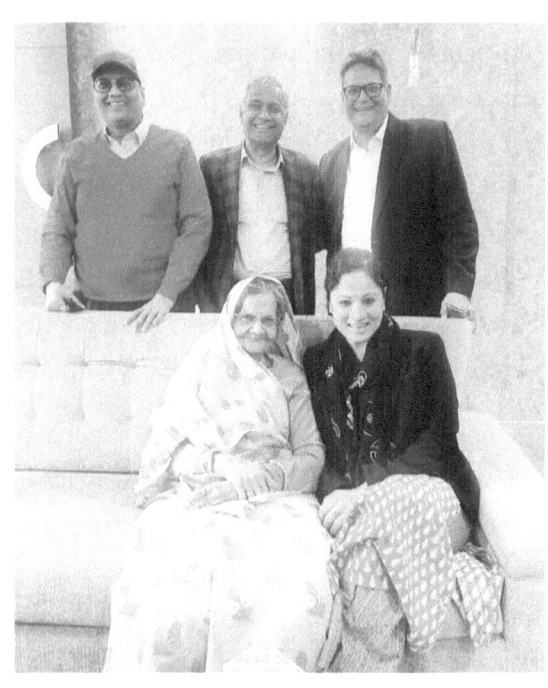

My only sister, Rajul and brother-in-law, Vinod JI, also came from Bengaluru to see me. I observed that Rajul was trying her best to hide her tears while sitting with me and holding my hands as a loving younger sister would do in such a situation. Her mere presence has given me motivation and uplifted my overall temperament. I understood that Vinod Ji was getting updates about me and my test results. He was also talking to Harsh about my treatment and well-being. He was very concerned about my illness and hoped for a speedy recovery. Rajul along with her daughter, Priyanka, who is a specialist in pranic healing, put in the extra effort to travel frequently to Delhi from Bengaluru to take care of my health and comfort me during my treatment. Her calming nature and optimistic attitude always lifted my spirits.

My nephew, Rishabh and his wife, Aanchal took great care of me during my entire stay in Delhi and very carefully managed all my needs during the entire period of my treatment despite the COVID pandemic that was at its peak in India. They regularly played cards and other games with me to help me stay in a good mood. They ensured that I was safe and secure by not allowing anyone coming from outside to directly step into my room. Rishabh's sons, Arihant and Shaurya, both brothers used to come to my room very often and play with me and Suman. I do like to play with children, and I also have some fond memories of playing with adults when I was a child. I actually think most adults enjoy playing with children if they figure out the games that fit everyone's abilities and interests.

My niece, Dr. Noopur Jain, who is a renowned dermatologist and her husband, Dr. Ankit Jain who is also a plastic surgeon has been like pillars of support to me. I must admit that it was a blessing that Dr. Ankit was working in Medanta Hospital—the same hospital where I was being treated. He took extraordinary care of me and ensured that I had no discomfort while being injected with chemo. It was he who coordinated with all the doctors and nursing staff of different departments during the entire period of my treatment. He always went the extra mile to make things easier for me. I will always thank God for making such a nice person a part of our family.

My eldest nephew, Deepak, was visibly disturbed when he came to meet me along with his wife, Vineeta. They were both so concerned that their faces were telling the story of the pain they felt for me.

My nieces, Jyoti and her husband, Vikas Ji and Pratibha and her husband, Sunny Ji, were all with me when I visited Mumbai and took great care of coordinating all the logistics and needs for all of us there.

My sister-in-law, Mausam and her husband, Abhinav, visited me regularly from Gurgaon to check on my health and spent a lot of time with me.

My exceptional gratitude to my mother-in-law, Smt. Ratni Devi, who despite her old age, came to see and bless me. My brother-in-law, Bhagchand ji, Sumitra Bhabi and Rajendra Ji who despite his illness came along with his wife, Suman, to see me several times to give me moral support.

My special gratitude goes to my elder daughter-in-law, Shilpa's parents, Mahendra Ji and his wife, Sarita who frequently visited me and gave me valuable moral support. My younger daughter-in-law, Priyanshi's parents, Pawan Ji Didwania and Alka Ji and her Uncle and Aunt Anupam ji and Sonal visited me frequently. They supported me during my meetings with the doctors and gave me moral support, for which I will always be indebted.

Each member of my family played a very important role in strengthening my resolve to overcome the disease. Throughout my treatment, everyone supported me. They insisted that if I could overcome so many hurdles and challenges previously in my life, I had the strength to do so now too.

The line by Lee Iacocca reminds me of the true value of a family:

"The only rock I know that stays steady, the only institution I know that works, is the family."

My eldest grandson, Yuvan, all of 10 years now is a very good cricketer. During a tournament organised by my company, he was the youngest player to win a 'Man of the Match' trophy for his exemplary bowling and taking the wickets of some of the good players. Despite being so young, he has been showing mature behaviour and I can see a great man in the making. He always has an aura of determination and undoubtedly, his presence has always stoked strong will in everyone, including me.

Sanaya is a soft and sensitive girl. Though she is just 7 years old, her nature of sharing and caring is prevalent in all her activities.

I had always loved and enjoyed having ice-creams with my grandchildren. It had been quite a regular affair in the past, however, after my treatment, I had altogether stopped having sweets and ice cream. One day, when I was at home, my 3 grandkids wanted to have an ice cream party and had ordered Chocobars. Sanaya, along with her brothers, Yuvan and little Riaan, came together holding ice-creams in their hands and there was one for me as well.

On informing them that I had stopped eating ice cream, Sanaya was so taken aback that she continued looking at me unaware that her own ice cream was melting. Before she could realise this, it got detached from the stick and fell. She looked at the fallen piece of ice cream and then looked at me and started sobbing. Her innocence had surfaced through every tear in her eyes. It was a shock for them that their dearest companion, *Dadu*, would no longer have any ice cream with them.

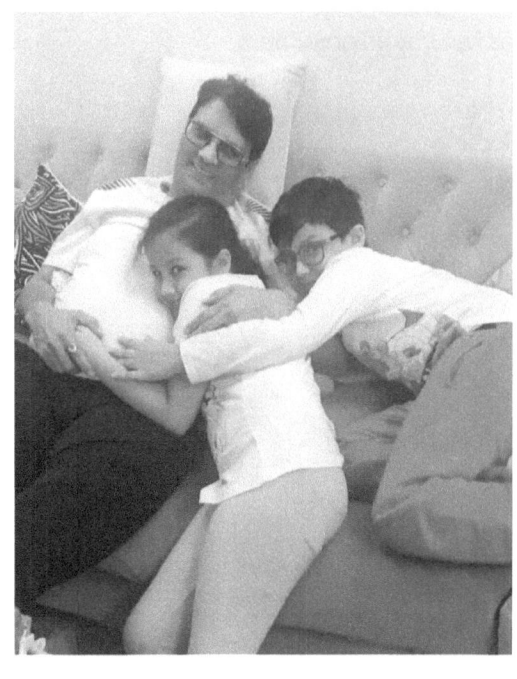

Kids are so innocent to accept the changes in life. For them, love is always unadulterated and not tarnished by the ravages of time.

Everyone says that during the crests and troughs of every human life, the family is the 'pillar of rock' and I can proudly say that for my whole family. I was overwhelmed by their unconditional love, care and support. I have always thanked God for giving me such a loving and beautiful family.

A beautiful line by Elizabeth Jane Howard in her book, *Families* signifies the importance of a family. She has written: "Call it a clan, call it a network, call it a tribe, call it a family: whatever you call it, whoever you are, you need one."

Surrounded by my family and well-wishers I never thought about the outcome. Instead, I tried using my energy to focus on my wellness and what I can do to make life more interesting and stay as healthy as possible.

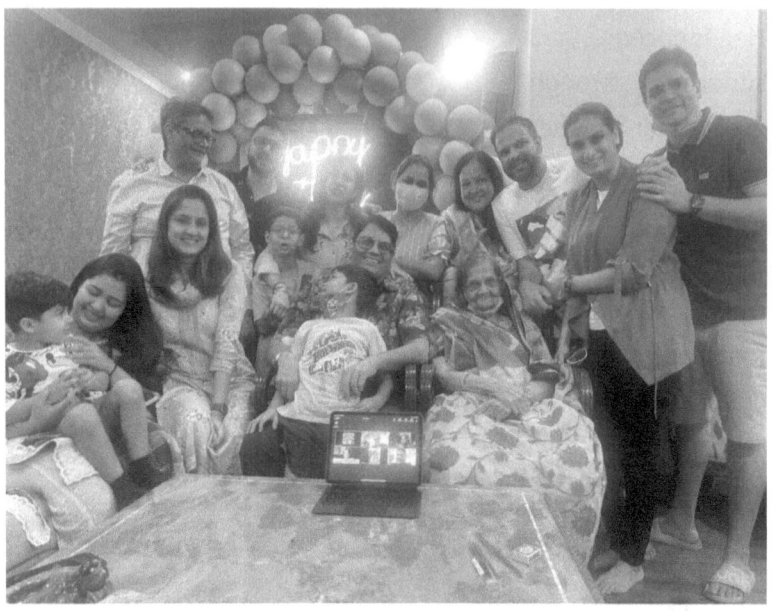

Life has taught me to look for positives in every situation. Sometimes this means looking for the good even during times that are harsh and trying to be hopeful instead of thinking about the worst.

Key Takeaways:

- When suffering from difficult diseases, always seek the opinion of several specialists. Never rush for treatment based on a single diagnosis report.
- Sweets, white flour, and packaged foods should be avoided as much as possible.

- Always try to have a systematic approach to life. Create systems that work well for you.
- Communication should be clear and proper. Medical practitioners and even common people should be humane in their communication with patients and their families.
- Chemotherapy reduces the immunity of the body. A person undergoing it should avoid travelling between successive sessions of chemotherapies.
- Even during the worst of times, never surrender to fear. Remember, there are ways to solve a problem and that always works.
- Always try to be upbeat and energetic. It lifts the spirits of people close to you.

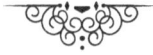

PHASE 3
RECOVERY

THE ROAD TO RECOVERY

One of the famous lines on cancer I have read so far is from the book *Live On* by Fabi Powell. He has written, "When cancer happens, you don't put life on hold. You live now."

My brother-in-law, Rajendra Jain, is quite close to me. In fact, for the last 20 years, he has been my travelling partner to several destinations. My first ever encounter with cancer was when I stayed with him in Gurgaon for his treatment of cancer at Medanta. It was a time of peak COVID infection and so, we did not allow others to join us during the course of the treatment. This whole episode impacted me greatly and even altered my way of looking at life.

In my extended family, nobody has ever been diagnosed with cancer until the year 2020 when my brother-in-law, Rajendra Jain, was affected by the disease. During his treatment, I was there to spend time with him. I had seen his resolve to confront the intruder and emerge victorious. I witnessed his pain, struggle and grit but I never imagined then that the roles would reverse so quickly. However, knowing the various steps and processes of the treatment helped me a lot when it was detected.

He was diagnosed with throat cancer and the doctors advised him to undergo an operation but they also cautioned that the operation might have adverse effects on him and he may lose his voice. So, instead of living a life without a voice, he decided not to get operated. We then consulted many doctors across the world who had voiced the same opinion.

The alternative was to go through the process of radiation he was administer 35 doses of the same. This was the right decision as he recovered from the disease.

As I have witnessed the value of thorough research and consultations for different forms of treatment in his and my case, I would suggest that the patient and his relatives research extensively for the type of ailment. They can go through data that is easily available on the internet and other online platforms. They also need to consult different specialists instead of making hasty decisions regarding their treatment methods.

I had seen him struggle during his radiation sessions. He required support to even get up and walk. He had told me that his legs felt like a mass of jelly with no bones or strength. He explained to me that nothing was painless through the process but the struggle helped to keep the mind strong. Taking help for mundane activities is always embarrassing.

No matter how much you try, negative thoughts always linger in the mind. It becomes worse when one frets and worries about the future. There are innumerable blessings that need to be counted rather than ruining over mistakes, disappointments or missed chances. Staying positive creates a unique strength within. I have witnessed that in my brother-in-law. His aura of positivity never diminished through the courses of treatment and recovery. I too tried to emulate him and it has worked well for me.

There have been times when I felt helpless, lonely, and anxious. However, these lines from a life coach, Rachelle Triay, gave me strength and boosted my morale.

In her book, she has written, "When the road gets hard, do not quit. When you are unsure of your next steps, pray and seek counsel, then keep moving." By shutting myself off from the past and future, I was able to improve my positive mental framework. Sometimes, it saddened me or even made me feel guilty for infusing anxiety and fear into the minds of people who loved me. When my brother-in-law came to meet me, I had a feeling that he would offer doses of wisdom to help me cope with my current situation.

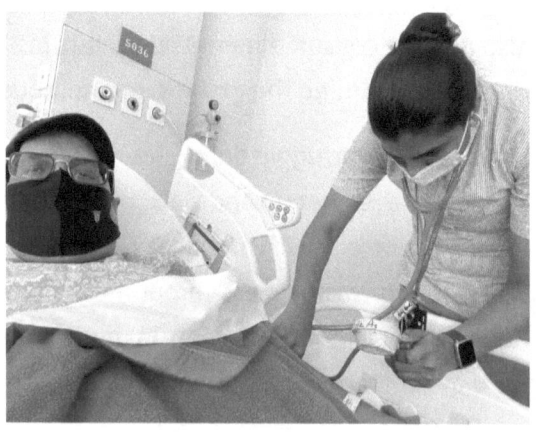

However, we chatted about everything other than cancer that day. We even joked and laughed at various issues that ranged from business and politics to sports and cinema. I was amazed at the fact that this man had been struggling to manage himself a year ago and here he was, cheerful and full of life. I realized why he did not give me any advice. His presence in front of me was enough. It made me realize that no ailment can suppress the will to live and no advice is needed for the one who can stay positive within oneself. That visit strengthened my resolve by several notches and helped me regain the upper hand in my fight against the disease.

Chemo brought with it senses of drowsiness, nausea and a feeling of intense warming up of the veins. I was weakened by the 6 doses of strong chemotherapy, so I restricted myself from all non-essential movements and activities. The side effects of chemo had started to show and I had to fight out regular attacks of nausea, exhaustion and other discomforts. Even though I was shrouded in weakness, I had irregular sleep patterns. If the chemo sessions were like wrestling bouts, the aftermath was more like a boxing match.

However, my indomitable nature always prompted me to get up every time and face reality head-on. I had faith in myself and believed that I could rebound after every storm that comes my way.

While affected by cancer, I came to know that the human body and mind have extraordinary powers that are always taken for granted. If one is receptive to these powers, the human mind and body can bring about immense courage to withstand pain and depression. The treatment and recovery phases come with their own set of challenges. It is time to unlearn and relearn.

During my chemo sessions, it was a rendezvous with the unknown. As I lay each time for the process, looking silently at the dripping chemical being infused into my bloodstream, my mind wondered how the sentinels would deal with the intruders who lay deep within the cell structure.

Most of the doctors, nurses and caregivers appeared nonchalant through the procedures since such scenes were daily affairs for them. However, a few were concerned and friendly. One nurse often visited me, sometimes even out of turn. A few times, I had seen utter amazement in her eyes, seeing my resilience. Sometimes, I joked with her and talked about my family and hobbies.

"You are different from the other patients," she used to say. This was something I already knew. I had watched other patients who seemed crestfallen, as if having surrendered themselves to the inevitable. However, my internal chemistry had always been greater than my external physics. I always held on to my obstinate zeal to come out of even the trickiest of situations and never let external pressures get the best of me.

One day, while I was waiting at the chemo lounge, I managed to sneak in a few jokes with my wife and other family members. A few others were also around. But unlike the other morose characters, I appeared to be the most upbeat. The nurse got curious. She dropped her half-finished coffee into the bin and approached me.

"Sir, you are about to receive one of the strongest chemical concoctions today. I am surprised that you are so enthusiastic right before this."

It was quite unexpected of her to ask me that question, as she has seen a number of patients being stressed and scared before their medical procedure. I told her, "My dear, life is about living the moment. If you allow gloom to overcome you, it is an act of betrayal that you commit against those who are praying and hoping for your recovery."

The nurse looked stunned.

"Yes, sir. I have experienced it and am now content with my present," she said.

Slowly but steadily, I developed a bond with the hospital staff. They had been equally enthusiastic and curious about seeing me jovial and upbeat every time and I never disappointed them. Dealing with gloomy-faced patients may have annoyed them. But seeing me with a smiling face made them lively and active. There are methods to recover from the downward syndrome. Being prepared for pain reduces it. The ability to think one step after the other allows you to walk without support. Thinking about the blessings and the brighter side of life subdues bouts of depression. Taking deep breaths and keeping a relaxed mind fights nausea and having an unwavering faith in God eases the brain of all worries and uncertainty. I was indeed lucky to have a group of loving people around me and that made things much easier. Your mother and wife are the two most affected people by every hiccup in life. I was lucky to always have both of them by my side.

I also developed an affinity for some of the most dedicated hospital staff. However, I was worried about developing Stockholm syndrome (Stockholm syndrome is a condition in which hostages develop a psychological bond with their captors during captivity).

This term came into being in 1973 when four people were taken hostage by bank robbers in Stockholm, Sweden. After their release, the hostages were adamant about not testifying against their captors in court. They had somehow grown fond of the captors instead of treating them with fear, disdain and vengeance.

A doctor's touch is one of the most important aspects of healing a patient, as it works as a reassuring gesture. I remember once hearing a lecture by an eminent cardiologist, Dr. Devi Shetty, about the importance of touching a patient and how and why a doctor should do it. The emotional quotient associated with the touch of a doctor adds essential confidence and belief in a patient. I have experienced this wonder and would like to solicit all doctors to do so. This little humane action brings about a lot of comfort and is instrumental in lifting the morale of the patient and their kith and kin. It is also necessary for the patient to be communicative and not be retracted into a shell. Suffering in silence worsens the situation. To keep your mind free from negative thoughts, it's helpful to engage in meaningful discussions with others. This keeps your mind unburdened and prevents morbid thoughts from creeping in.

There were many people in the hospital who had grown fond of me too. One such person was a ward boy who always carried the various instruments for my chemo sessions. He was always there beside the bed to recline it or make any other adjustments as per the comfort of the patient. He was a cheerful lad and quite often liked to engage in short discussions with me. These discussions often calmed my nerves and helped me relax and undergo the process with ease.

If you look at it, a chemo session seems simple to describe. You start with one of the most mandatory steps—signing a few papers that describe all the side effects one can acquire after the process. It is a protocol that cannot be skipped. After these formalities, the patient is allowed to go back and prepare themselves. This involves more psychological conditioning than physical in order to be prepared for the processes that will be done the next day. I must admit that the day before a chemo session is indeed a very tough one. Today, talking about it, I feel comfortable enough because the moment, like any other, has turned into a memory.

If the treatment was a war, the process of recovery was no less than a series of small battles. My body was facing the impact of high-potency chemicals. This was challenging my normal routines, even my food and liquid intake. I decided to feed my body all fresh and unadulterated food and drinks and I completely switched to organic, unprocessed food, fruits and vegetables. I also stopped watching news, horror and fiction shows on TV or reading about violence or negativity. I loved walking on the grass, doing meditation and listening to the soulful chants of *Strotra Bhaktamar,* and other devotional mantras.

My consciousness seemed to bring me closer to God. However, I stayed secluded. In order to bring my body back to the required level of immunity, I had to stay away from some people and places. That gave me a lot of time to self-analysing what was needed to have a fulfilling life. It is paramount to actually know oneself. There is a stark contrast between loneliness and solitude. Loneliness is a negative attribute, where you are left with no choice as a result of people tending to

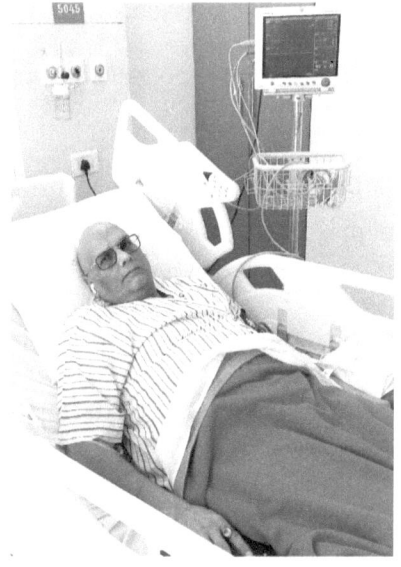

stay away from you. Solitude is more of a choice to remain with oneself.

It provides us with information about ourselves, that generally, we tend to be ignorant of. When we get ourselves immersed in work, we hardly get time to think about or know about ourselves. Knowing oneself is the greatest knowledge one can acquire. Solitude gives us the time to do so. With every possible precautionary measure for the body and mind, I managed to ride over all the discomforts that chemo brings about. Initially, whenever I looked in the mirror, I was disgusted with the reflection of my puffy face and shaven head. However, as time passed, I grew accustomed to this and came to accept it as my 'new look.'

Whenever I was bored or felt my days were monotonous, I recalled some famous anecdotes of *Akbar and Birbal* to lift my spirits. One such story of Birbal's wisdom comes to mind.

Once, Akbar and Birbal were strolling in the palace gardens. Suddenly, Akbar asked a weird question to catch Birbal off guard.

He asked, "Can you tell me how many crows are there in our kingdom?"

Birbal was spontaneous in his answer, "Your Majesty, there are eighty thousand nine hundred and seventy-one crows in our kingdom."

Surprised, Akbar further probed, "What if we have more crows?"

Birbal replied, "Oh, then the crows from the other kingdoms must be visiting us."

"What if there are lesser crows?" asked Akbar.

"Well, then some of our crows must be visiting their relatives in other kingdoms," replied Birbal promptly. Akbar had no answer to Birbal's presence of mind.

My stay in Delhi has allowed me to read more amusing, interesting and thoughtful stories from Akbar-Birbal, Panchtantra, etc. It kept me amused and also brought back happy childhood memories. Though I had no official work, my days were busy. I did yoga, meditation, listened to devotional songs, read meaningful quotations and watched motivational videos and in between managed to have a few hours of rest.

I could feel that I was healing! But was I?

EMERGING OUT OF UMBRA

I have read a quote somewhere by Robert Alden that said, "There is not enough darkness in all the world to put out the light of even one small candle."

It was the 7th day after my last chemotherapy when I along with Suman, Harsh and Shilpa went to see Dr. Ashok Vaid to share with him my full test reports and PET scan findings. After looking at the reports, the doctor announced that I was left with no cancerous cells but I would have to wait to proclaim myself "cancer-free."

It was an unexpected remark from my doctor. I was perplexed as to what could be the reason behind this advice to wait before proclaiming myself free from the disease. Is there any other method that will determine the cure of cancer? Some thoughts of radiation came to mind as I was aware of it in 2020 itself when my brother-in-law, Rajendra Jain was advised to get the doses of radiation. So, I took the chance and asked my doctor whether radiation would be required in my case too. The doctor looked undecided for some time before instructing me to go for radiation. His advice was not very convincing to us and I also knew that radiation brought with it more perils. Hence, we decided to get opinions from different specialists before making any further plans.

Even though some of the contacts in India made the same suggestion, we still felt the need for more scouting. I have started firmly believing in the fact that while deciding upon the treatment for a deadly disease, one should always take multiple opinions and not be in haste. So, we got in touch with the doctors from abroad for some elaborate explanation.

An oncologist from Singapore, who had looked extremely affable and conceptually strong, aired a different view. He pointed out that radiation is dangerous for the affected region because it may damage the esophagus and the vocal cord. This is something no other oncologist has pointed out. After consultation amongst ourselves and a couple of discussions with the same specialist, we decided to refrain from radiation. We felt that this was the right suggestion at the right moment.

We consulted another oncologist from the Mayo Hospital, USA on this matter and they also echoed the same suggestion that I do not go for the radiation treatment.

> During the whole period of my recovery, I never missed out on any festival or celebration. During these testing times, I realized that we have one life and it should be lived to the fullest.

Though the pall of gloom had almost lifted knowing that treatment had come to an end, I did not indulge in any overt celebration. It was a new lease of life for me and it was time to thank God and all the people who had stayed with me in support throughout the darkest period of my life.

It is a fact that the fear of the unknown is sometimes overwhelming. However, something that makes it look surmountable is the leap of faith. My faith in myself and my team's faith in a positive outcome made it easy for me to come out unscathed. Early detection and diagnosis of cancer is essential for the success of the treatment. People need to be made aware of the early signs of cancer and when and how to get checked. This is the sole motto of the Indian Cancer Society. I was lucky to have detected the disease early in time and thus, I am able to return to a normal life today. However, the recovery period gave me time to soak up in all the learning and lessons that I believe one should learn from life. Though there might be many people around the world with the highest degrees in academics, the teachings of life are indeed paramount.

Though I was with my loved ones in Delhi, at times I felt pangs of longing for my city, Kolkata. This was a time when the city got into a festive mood. Though COVID had imposed a lot of restrictions, the people were hard to contain. Every year in August, the essence of *Durga Puja* (a famous Hindu festival) begins to drift in the air. A true resident of Bengal will always look for the dates of *Durga Puja* in a calendar and I was no exception to this ritual. It is always a time to meet old friends in the city and spend quality time with family and relatives. The sound of *"Dhak"* (drum beat) envelopes the air and people could be seen pandal (marquee) hopping in colorful attires. Sometimes, I felt that I missed the fervor of my city.

Like all metropolis around the world, Kolkata has a life of its own. It has a heart throbbing with art, literature, music and culture. I had been fortunate to be familiar with the most virtuous contemporaries of the city and some from the past as well. My association with various clubs and organizations in Kolkata has always allowed me to be in close proximity to some famous and talented names in this part of the country. However, I had learned to adapt to situations exceedingly well. My foremost priority was to recover completely and hence, I did not mind being in Delhi.

Home-sickness is a behavioral disorder that is mainly found in students and workers who get posted far from home and this emotion often brings about negative feelings. Many a time, I have counseled my employees not to feel dejected if they get posted to remote locations. Most of the projects that my business executes are usually located in places that are far from cities. Of course, a lack of proper facilities may hurt at times but it is always beneficial to adapt to the conditions as quickly as possible.

Home-sickness causes unnecessary sorrow and drooping shoulders never yield productivity. The best method is to live and enjoy the present moment and not yearn for the past. I had made Delhi my home and had started loving every little thing that came my way. It didn't matter whether it was a walk along the balcony, a stroll in the green grass below or gazing endlessly at the flowers in the garden; everything brought about a sense of awe.

However, my longing for Kolkata had other reasons too. I missed my grandchildren and pets a lot. They have always given me immense joy and provided me with pleasurable hours of relaxation. My grandchildren visited me in Delhi with their parents a few times.

Yet, I sorely missed being with them regularly. My two Labradors, Bailey and Brandy, were very fond of me. It pained me to think how they might have been missed my presence.

My mind told me that I had recovered from my ailment, but the lingering fear of a relapse always haunted my thoughts. Harsh had been searching for solutions to eliminate the chances of a relapse. He had conducted online consultations with several doctors across the globe to understand the situation that I was in. All the doctors from abroad whom we had consulted had given us patient hearings, which had soothed our nerves to a great extent. I am indeed grateful to some of the foreign doctors who spent a good amount of time listening to us patiently and giving valuable advice. Their courteous and attentive hearing was heartening and in fact, the manner in which each doctor corresponded with us with clarity provided us the confidence.

During the process of my treatment, I learned that one of the prime areas of effective medical treatment is proper communication. Professionals in western countries are conducting advanced research on the various methodologies in patient care. How to touch a patient or speak to a patient, and how to break serious news to the patient or their relatives are all important for medical practitioners to know. In fact, every person needs to know the right way to communicate different types of news, especially if it is of a serious nature. Death is something that has a lot of emotions attached to it. Even though we all know that death is imminent and a looming reality, the fear of death and the emotions attached to it will always remain prevalent. Of course, there are exceptions to this.

It can be difficult to know what to say to someone with cancer. Unless you've been there yourself, you can't possibly understand how it feels. Years ago, people spoke in whispers about cancer. Today, even with the widespread availability of treatment and improved chances of survival, numerous individuals remain uncertain about how to cope with such news. There should be some rules of conduct or etiquette for communicating with a cancer patient or survivor. I will be describing it in detail in the chapter 'Cancer Etiquette' for readers to understand what could be the right approach to talk with a person already under the burden of the disease.

Many cancer survivors share similar stories that detail awkward encounters and upsetting comments made by well-meaning individuals. Their collective observations help us define 'cancer etiquette,' or rules of conduct for communicating with the cancer community. Since each person's experience with cancer is different, one approach does not necessarily work for everyone.

One of my close friends in Mizoram had lost his only son who was just in his early thirties. Since I happened to be close to the family, I was deeply aggrieved by the news. However, when I visited him with teary eyes, I was surprised by his demeanor.

He said, "Why are you crying? God had given me a son and it was His prerogative to take him back. We always go back to our source and my son too has gone back to his source." The maturity of his thoughts absolutely stumped me. If everyone were to adopt this way of thinking, most of their stress that pertains to death could be significantly diminished.

The limited number of people, apart from my family members who knew about my plight, were also eager to know about my recovery. My chauffeurs who had always been my strong supporters were inquiring about my whereabouts and were in tears to know that I was yet to recover. It was unadulterated love. When such messages reached me, I was overwhelmed by emotions. I had to recover fast for myself, my family and all the people who loved and prayed for me. I knew people longed to see me as the person I was before being diagnosed with cancer—busy working and committed to projects. I felt that I had changed but for the better. In fact, there is a reason why cancer is called the 'tsunami disease.'

When a tsunami comes, it breaks all old and weak structures, while shaking the stronger ones as well. It also brings new vegetation and soil with it. Similarly, this disease also wipes out weak and unclear mindsets and replaces them with clear and vibrant thoughts. The disease had brought about several changes in me too. I am now more resolute, caring and spiritual. I learned the value of my wellbeing, not only physically, but mentally, socially and spiritually as well.

So here I was—a changed person, embedded and enriched by the lessons of life—ready to embark on a fresh start. I longed to get into my new phase of life and spread all the knowledge I had acquired to those who needed it the most. I wanted to spread the message of positivity in the ensuing negative atmosphere. I wanted to belong to the masses once more—to be part of the sprawling vastness of the country with hooting trains, crying cars, shouting buses, ribbons of roads, wandering people, chaotic lifestyles, ignorant patients, and mindless advisors to assert the value that life presented.

I wanted to shout out to people that they needed to love life and be happy with their present dispositions. I wanted to soothe the disillusioned teenagers of their needless sorrow and assure them of better times that lie ahead.

The decision not to undergo radiation brought an overwhelming sense of relief, marking the completion of my treatment. As entire family gathered together, a feeling of comfort and gratitude enveloped us, knowing I had reached this stage. The past six months replayed like a movie in our minds. We decided to fly back home very next day. With a rejuvenated spirit, I went to bed that night, with my mind at peace.

During that night, a vivid dream occurred. My father appeared, holding my hands as if guiding me towards a new life ahead. He bestowed upon me words of wisdom and blessings. The next morning, I woke up with a newfound determination to embrace my new life with even more passion.

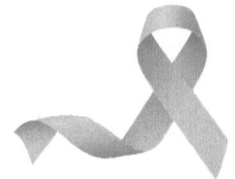

BACK TO THE CITY OF JOY

There are many stories of cancer survivors. Some of these depict the strength and resilience of these people. This truly is inspiring and gives the person hearing it a new source of energy and enthusiasm. I had read about Douglas Clarke who was a firefighter in America. He was diagnosed twice with cancer—first with lung cancer and then it reached to his brain. In spite of these challenges, Douglas continued to fight fires, and taught about the fire safety.

He once said, "I won't let cancer define me, but I'll use my journey to help others."

I fully believed his words and was fixed on not letting cancer define my future. I am sure my efforts to make my experience known to others will inspire other cancer patients to fight with courage and make life post-treatment more fulfilling.

With great enthusiasm and a newfound energy, my family and I landed at Kolkata airport. A feeling of excitement and anticipation filled the air as we embarked on our journey in this vibrant city. The drive back home was exceedingly exciting. I felt like a child coming back home from the hostel after a long time. Sometimes, I craned my neck to see the changes that had come about in the city.

Was the overhead metro running? Were there new hotels, clubs, and stores? The best thing about Kolkata is that it is not a very huge city but it also houses some of the most pristine clubs that guarantee wonderfully relaxed evenings with family and friends.

As the car neared my home, I felt the old emotions of the city flooding me. Memories do not have expiry dates. Everybody had gathered to welcome me. My grandchildren were especially overjoyed to have me back with them. I have always cherished their company and enjoyed the innocent questions they often come up with. They asked me with similar barrages of questions in a rapid or overwhelming manner. My long absence must have increased their curiosity.

My Labradors, Belly and Brandy, whom I badly missed in Delhi, did not come close to me initially. Perhaps, they thought I was someone else because of my shaven head. Time and again, they looked at me from a distance in utter disbelief, which was evident in their eyes. However, dogs have some extraordinary perceptions.

After some time, both the dogs could recognize me and were elated by the discovery. They simply leapt at me in joy and licked my feet and face to say that they too missed me. They would not stop wagging their tails and sometimes, they let out low growls as if complaining about my long absence. This is the type of unadulterated love that cannot be overlooked.

Despite my family members advising me not to spend time with the pets for a while, to stay away from any infections, their love for me and the joy of seeing and recognizing me couldn't be ignored. They wouldn't leave me even for a short while and kept pouring their love through various activities. These are the ingredients of happiness. Life is more enjoyable and exciting for us when we come to know about feelings, emotions and happiness through our own discoveries.

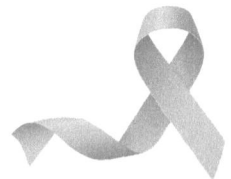

MOMENTS TO CHERISH

Rachelle Triay, a life coach has meaningfully said, "You only have one today, one tomorrow. You only have one life. Let's make the most of it. Let's choose to grow!"

The turbulent times I went through created a new belief system in me. I realized that this episode of my life had made me learn a lot about life. Today, I know that life is not about ruining the past or fretting about the future. It is about living and enjoying the present!

Being with myself in solitude enabled me to understand myself better. I had learned about quite a few attributes of myself that I had been unaware of. It made me truly realize the value of taking life easy and enjoying every moment that we are blessed with.

It felt a little strange without board meetings, paperwork, client visits, official agendas, office protocols, project reviews, etc. But I used that time to connect with myself and re-discover the person I am.

There are so many positives that life has brought about during this period.

My mother who still calls me by my nickname, has always been anxious regarding my situation. She felt restless for not seeing me during my chemo sessions, even though we resided at the same place. I was not allowed to go out of my room since my immunity was low and the fear of an infection was high. One day, despite her knee problem I could hear her climbing the stairs 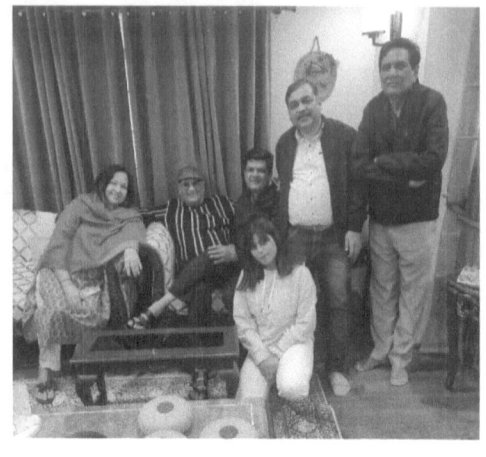 slowly. Just to see me from a distance, she took a lot of time and effort. It made me realize the strength of a mother's love, which is a powerful medicine and can cure any disease. I am a living example to prove that. Her love and care are something so important to me that they have been engraved in my mind.

Before my detection of cancer, we three brothers and one sister did not talk to each other frequently because of our individual work pressures and whenever we talked it was concerning business activities only. However, my illness has given us a chance to grow closer and bond. Now, we talk almost every day and most of our topics are bereft of business. Much like a few years ago, we have planned to meet once a year with our families and spend quality time together. But the best thing that happened after my full recovery was that we siblings, along with our spouses went on a trip to Port Blair and stayed there and thoroughly enjoyed our long-awaited reunion.

During adverse times, one can test if their friends are true and dedicated. When things are bright, a lot of people might come in to contact with you and remain friendly. However, when you are going through a dark phase, only your true companions and family members stay in touch and support you.

There are innumerable contacts on everyone's mobile phones. I feel that from these contacts, one should identify a minimum of 20 contacts whom they can truly consider their best well-wishers. They can be family members, friends or even office colleagues. They are the ones who will stand by you like a rock in your difficult times. While dealing with them, always use your heart and not your head. I mean to say that try to ignore small frictions and accept them. If needed make the necessary adjustments or compromises with them. They are the people who will help and support you when you need them the most. I have done the same and I also urge all to do it as well. You may call them whatever group you wish to, as I have saved all their names with the prefix 'farishte' (angels).

> I realized that anything can happen to anyone at any point of time. There have been many cases where a seemingly healthy person has fallen prey to COVID and passed away. So, it is advisable to sometimes consciously slow down and enjoy every moment.

The world around us is becoming more and more violent and selfish. To thrive in this atmosphere of negativity, one must remain positive. The unprovoked atrocities in Ukraine are a reminder. That's why throughout my treatment I have tried to be very positive and always looked at the brighter side of things. This outlook helped me cope with this disease. I have realized that without the support of my loved ones, it would have been too difficult to remain optimistic and strong.

I also realized that whenever somebody meets patients who are suffering from such a fateful disease, they should encourage them to share their feelings. It does not matter if you are a friend, a family member or just a well-wisher. All you need is to assert your allegiance with a gentle pat on the back, laughter or offering a simple hug, as we call them *Jaadu ki Jhappi*. You could lend your ear to hear them out but try to refrain from trying to advise them. A person who is suffering from such a disease is sure to be overwhelmed with feelings of hopelessness and loneliness. At such a point in time, if we can show genuine love, care and compassion, it can do wonders for them and will go a long way to curing them.

I feel blessed to know some people have postponed important engagements to be with me. I feel all the more lucky to see how happy they are knowing that I have successfully fought and been declared free from the disease. This will remain in the happy alcoves of memory. From here on, I made a promise to myself that I would not miss out on any event, festival or family gathering on the pretext of being busy. Every occasion is a once-in-a-lifetime opportunity. Happiness is precious and it does not come with only material acquisitions. It comes through the feeling of being loved, treasured and thought of.

I have observed that many people prioritise monetary resources above other things. I feel that it doesn't deserve to be held on such a high pedestal but I have also realized why they do so. For example, let's create two different lists: one is a list of things that money can buy that will bring happiness and the other list contains things that money cannot buy but will still bring happiness. I am sure that the second list of what money cannot buy will be much bigger than the first list of what money can buy.

Money can buy the best of the property, but it does not have the power to convert it into a home.

Money can buy branded clothes and the best of jewellery, but it does not have the power to give you beauty and smartness.

Money can give you the best of healthcare, but it does not have the power to give you good health.

Money can buy you good food, but it does not have the power to provide you with a good digestive system.

Money can buy the most comfortable bed, but it does not have the power to give you a good sleep.

One can find many things that money can't buy. If money were the sole criterion for happiness and contentment, then many internationally acclaimed celebrities and film stars would not have committed suicide or died at an early age. Money can be used to buy anything in the world but there is no shop where you can walk and buy happiness and so, it is very clear that money can't buy happiness.

I had been advised by the doctors to take good care of my body and have a checkup done after a few months. This time, I was sure that nothing would come in my way of complete recovery and that I would come out with flying colors. I kept up with the strict regimen of diet, meditation and positive thinking and realized that I was improving in all dimensions. Besides my physical transformation as a result of hair loss, I also changed myself mentally, emotionally and spiritually. The new "me" spread a lot of happiness and I appeared to be immensely confident.

It is always a blessing to have a loving family stick with you through thick and thin. Nowadays, the concept of a joint family has become almost antiquated. However, having an extended family together gives person a lot of strength. We should always be thankful to God for providing us with meaningful relationships. One of the best feelings in the world is to make someone happy with your compliments. We might thank strangers countless times for doing a small favor or providing us with small bits of help. But how many times do we stop to thank our parents, spouses, children, siblings or members of an extended family or even our support staff? We generally, tend to take the good things in life for granted.

Today, when we are faced with multiple crises on earth, do we ever thank God for providing us with enough food, air, water and other natural resources? We have always taken them for granted and this has led to the deteriorating condition of this planet. Personally, I feel very happy and lucky because of the presence of my loved ones around me and also all the amenities I have had access to.

Whenever I thanked my wife, children, grandchildren, siblings or other loved ones, I felt unadulterated happiness from inside. The joy of making someone smile is priceless. It is worth the effort to compliment someone for the work they do to make your life comfortable. Even if the gardener, sweeper or driver get their salaries, when you compliment them for their work, you can feel the joy that they radiate. A positive atmosphere is one in which everyone feels wanted and loved. I feel that it is a dire necessity for each human being to create a positive ecosystem around them to sustain the precious life that they have been endowed with for centuries to come.

Sometimes, a simple line gives you solace in a challenging situation and asks you to be positive and optimistic.

Aaron Lauritsen has written in his book, a travelogue named *100 Days Drive: The Great North American Road Trip*, "There is strange comfort in knowing that no matter what happens today, the Sun will rise again tomorrow."

It sums up in the form to encourage us to follow our own path, chase our dreams, cherish what we have and liberate ourselves from needless worries.

INVALUABLE LIFE LESSONS

Many a time, I am compelled to think about why I got infected by cancer when I have always led a disciplined and healthy life. I have never fostered any ill habits or acquired any lifestyle disorders since my childhood. During various sessions of self-analysis, I could identify several points that had added to my learning about life. During my moments of solitude, I could recognize some aspects of life that we tend to live with.

When you are faced with difficult challenges, inspiring words, poems, messages or even watching videos can help soothe your nerves. I remember a few lines from Steve Maraboli's composition *Dare to Be*, which has always given me a new energy and enthusiasm:

> "When a new day begins, dare to smile gratefully.
>
> When there is darkness, dare to be the first to shine a light.
>
> When something seems difficult, dare to do it anyway.
>
> When life seems to beat you down, dare to fight back.
>
> When there seems to be no hope, dare to find some.

> When you're feeling tired, dare to keep going.
>
> When times are tough, dare to be tougher.
>
> Dare to be the best you can, at all times dare to be."

Sometimes, life surprises you by taking unexpected turns. It is important to be focused and grounded to sail through challenging phases. Everything passes. Good things, bad things, all things!

There are some relevant points that I would like to list out that need to be considered by everyone. Some of these attributes harm us and some help us on our journey through life.

The Dangerous World of Comparisons:

I had been comparing myself with others who had not been infected. This is something we keep doing throughout our lives and I have realized that it is wrong to do so. Everyone has a different journey. Some might be in a better position and some may be languishing in sorrow. However, comparisons never alleviate your condition. It rather adds to the feelings of self-pity and anxiety. These attributes are indeed harmful. It is vital that you are content and happy with what you have. Consider these blessings and cherish them.

Comparisons tend to belittle your capabilities and accomplishments. Unnecessary comparisons turn relationships bitter and sour the mind. People often create false impressions when they try to keep up with social comparisons. We have seen people go into depression because of unfair comparisons. Though the world today is more competitive, it is necessary to be happy with one's own possessions, which are generally taken for granted. We should admit to ourselves that we are privileged. In the illusionary world of comparisons, we end up harming ourselves much more in the long run.

You can be anything, but you can't be everything. When you compare yourself to others, you are basically comparing their best features against your average ones. It's like being right-handed and trying to play an instrument with your left hand and feeling bad about the result. Here, we are not only wanting to be better than the ones we compare ourselves with but the unconscious realization that we are not better than someone else, as a result of comparisons, becomes self-destructive.

Comparisons between people is a recipe for unhappiness unless you are the best in the world. Let's be honest, only one person can be the best of all. You may not be aware that others are probably comparing themselves to you—maybe you're better at your work, knowledge and experience than they are—and envious of you for various reasons. It is a fact that when we compare ourselves to others, we end up focusing our energy on bringing people down rather than raising ourselves up. We should not sabotage our happiness by ignoring the wonderful things in our lives.

> There is one thing that you're better at than other people—being you. This is the only game you can really master.

Life is all about being a better version of yourself, and when that happens, your effort and energy go towards upgrading your personal operating system every day and not worrying about what others are doing. This act of continuous development makes you happier and frees you from the shackles of false comparisons, allowing you to focus on the present moment.

What really matters is what you do, what your standards are and what you can actually learn and achieve. Every activity and thought goes through a process. Everyone's journey is different and so, comparisons actually give no meaning to life.

The most important things in life are measured internally. Thinking about what matters to you is hard. Playing to someone else's scoreboard is easy. That's why a lot of people do it. But winning the wrong game is pointless. You get one life. Play your own game.

Points to ponder:

- The most important things in life come from the inner self, not from the outside.
- Comparing yourself to others is a recipe for unhappiness.
- You can be anything, but you can't be everything.
- There is one thing that you're better at than other people: being you. This is the only game you can really win.
- Compare yourself to who you were yesterday and improve every day.
- Expectations are the bigger enemy of our happiness than our circumstances.

Many people fall prey to comparisons and end up making themselves unhappy. An unhappy mind falls prey to diseases quite easily. I have tried to reflect on whether I had ever fallen prey to the comparisons. It may or may not be the case. However, I know that now I am beyond any such emotion. I am surely not in the zone of comparison anymore. It does not even cross my mind.

The 26th President of the United States, Theodore Roosevelt, once said, "Comparison is the thief of joy." It steals away the joy and satisfaction from our lives.

There are so many things in life that we do not notice or often ignore. If we were to list five things for which we are grateful, we would notice all the things that we would have otherwise left unnoticed. This is my suggestion to understand how, sometimes, a simple thing that our mind does not pay attention to can, in reality, do wonders for the way we feel.

Stress: The Silent Killer

The era we live in is filled with stress and duress, making our lives all the more challenging. Every activity is accompanied by its inherent stress and punishing regimen. From school curriculums to work schedules, from travelling to socializing, everything comes with timelines and disciplines. Strain is embedded even in the mundane activities that we do and has become an integral part of our lives now. Furthermore, the world seems to be in a perennial hurry.

In education, career, sports, politics, finance, relationship, health and all other aspects of life, we have some degree of stress involved. Stress not only creates havoc with our health but also reduces human capacities like patience, forgiveness, gratitude, humility, endurance, empathy and love. The race to meet expectations is a mindless system that has now become a part of modern life. This race to meet has disturbed our balance between body, mind, and soul.

Satisfaction is not easy to attain, and the mind always remains unsettled. In our domain of business, i.e. EPC projects, we have a lot of competition and processes to deal with. Generally, the tenders are won by the L1 (lowest bidder) and that means the profit margins are very thin. The projects are spread over years and within the period of their execution, other problems may crop up. Even in the normal course, we are confronted by unfavorable weather, delays in approvals, local disputes or unrest, labor problems, shortages of materials, logistics and other issues.

However, we are required to deal with them all and complete the work within the statutory time period with no compromise on quality and design. The clients and consultants have a strict assessment, which keeps the team on their toes until the project is finished and handed over. Any delay, mistake or accident is dealt with strong measures which can result in heavy penalties or even termination of the contract. Sometimes, when we are engaged in simultaneous multi-dimensional projects, our engineering, execution and procurement team have to work long hours regularly to meet the deadlines.

It has been rightly said that 'turnover is vanity, profit is sanity and cash is reality'. Creating enough revenue to fund the company's growth is another stress. Over the years, our efforts have been met with remarkable success even though stress has always been part of the process. In our company, we make it a part of our training process to teach our people how to cope with stress.

Stress affects both the body and the brain. To maintain optimal mental and physical health, it is important to learn how to cope with stress.

I believe that the '5Ts Framework of Management' is a model that help guide the planning and execution of projects or other initiatives. It consists of five key elements that are crucial for successfully dealing with stress in life by a considerable margin.

> T1-Training: Training is required in all aspects of life. A properly trained person is an asset and can go a long way in fulfilling the responsibilities.
>
> T2-Technology: Sourcing the right technology is a matter of time. By using the right technology, one can eliminate human errors, complete a task faster and achive greater efficiency.
>
> T3-Timeliness: All activities should be time-bound. Otherwise, they create unnecessary backlogs. Timeliness allows work to flow seamlessly without much back-and-forth movement. It is this organized manner of working that yields better results.
>
> T4- Thought Process: The thought process of the entire team should be in sync with that of the management. The objectives of each employee should resonate with the mission, vision and value systems of the company. The management should also take care of the employees so that they always remain more energetic and loyal.
>
> T5- Team Building: Having a good and supportive team is the greatest asset for any captain. A good team always has players who can support each other, take on responsibilities and be held accountable. It is always more beneficial to have a good team than individual talents.

Even in our daily lives, stress has an overwhelming presence in mundane activities. Upon a closer inspection of various situations, we can understand that our own perceptions and assessments of situations are what lead to the development of stress. We fear the outcome of tomorrow and every result that may or may not come to our liking. Our fear and anxiety pressurize our minds. We need to accept our situations and think positively about the future. Live in the present, be your best self and be honest with your emotions. Life is ten percent what happens to us and ninety percent how we react to it. What lies behind us and what lies before us are tiny matters compared to what lies within us.

If the mind isn't kept under control, stress will keep getting into our system and keep triggering our fear for the future. I have experienced that whenever I get stressed for any reason, I tend to feel better if I take a few deep breaths and try to slow down my thought process. I try to think about the good things that have happened to me and fill my thoughts with gratitude for whatever I have achieved.

Stress is a dangerous ingredient to carry in life. Though we may not be able to do away with all the stress in our lives, we must try to keep it to a minimum level. It bodes well for our health. There are lots of coaches, mentors and gurus around the world who tell us about methods to diminish stress in our lives. Some of these discourses come from life experiences. It is worth listening to and learning from their experiences. During tough times, some of these lessons give us hope. I strongly believe that our problem is not the problem; our reaction to it is the real problem.

Negativity

The universe echoes the tune of the mind. While negativity gives rise to resentment, anger, anxiety and diseases, positivity is a miracle potion that heals. Life brings about its own share of happiness and gloom, but as per the law of attraction, one tends to attract what one chooses to think.

Negativity is a harbinger of ill health and a disturbed mind. It compels us to keep thinking about problems instead of searching for solutions. Every difficult situation brings with it a multitude of opportunities and only a positive mind can identify and benefit from them.

When one is sick, a lot of negative emotions run through the mind. During and after my process of healing and recovery, I always tried to focus on the positive aspects of life. When you search for cancer on the internet, a lot of worrisome and negative information emerges on the screen. I have stopped looking for more information about the disease. Instead, I look out for motivational speeches, soothing music and humor. I do not watch or read anything that depicts aggression or triggers negative emotions. It is possible that by sticking to a positive mental frame, I have been able to cure myself faster.

> For a life to be happy and fulfilled, one should have a positive attitude.

There is a story that I read in my childhood.

A man once told his grandchild that there were two creatures in every mind that were always in a tussle. One was evil and armed with anger, envy, greed, arrogance, violence and ego. The other was good and armed with peace, love, hope, empathy, gratitude and faith.

The kid asked his grandfather who the eventual winner was to which the grandfather told him that the one you feed more will eventually emerge stronger and win the fight. For life to be happy and fulfilled, one should have a positive attitude. It gives us a reason to enjoy our daily lives and to keep going when times are tough.

Social Networking

We have trained ourselves to thrive in virtual reality. Today, the world revolves around various social media platforms, which have become dominant players in modern society. All affirmations and negations in the form of symbols and comments have become the cardinal forces of life which is more of an illusion than authenticity. Currently, false information and miscommunication are prevalent in the world as a result of this. During the recent pandemic, a lot of false and misleading information was circulated through social media platforms. Instead of verifying such information, people accepted at face value and suffered immensely.

There can be no replacement of information from books and journals. However, social media has taught us to believe any post that we come across about history, geography, science, literature or even health issues. Digital media has made people lazy and even crazy. Solutions for simple mathematical calculations are also sourced from various devices. This has made the mind lose its alertness and become too dependent on external sources that may provide the wrong solution. For the past two decades, this new-age addiction has been prevalent, and if this trend continues to grow, the mental agility of future generations will suffer.

There is no better relaxation than reading. Replacing reading with online programs puts undue stress on the brain by making it process information at a faster pace. Rolling back to the good old habits of reading restores clarity of mind and our thoughts become more sensible.

Knowledge is Power

Knowledge is power, as it empowers people to know how to use the forces of nature for their benefit. We can differentiate between right and wrong, good and bad by employing our knowledge. I can say with conviction that knowledge is the pillar of success and good fortune.

Did you know that as per the Indian *Panchang* (calendar) system, each year which typically begins in mid-April has a specific name? And each name has a meaning! There are 60 names of years (*Samvatsars*). Each name repeats after 60 years.

The year 2019-20 was named 'Vikari' which lived up to its name by being a year filled with 'illness!'

The year 2020-21 was named 'Sharvari', meaning 'darkness' and it did push the world into a dark phase!

The 'Plava' year was 2021-22. 'Plava' means 'that which ferries us across.' The *Varaha Samhita* says: This will ferry the world across unbearable difficulties and take us to a state of glory, from darkness to light! (Varaha Samhita is an influential encyclopaedic text in Sanskrit that contains information on various topics such as astronomy, astrology, geography, architecture, weather forecasting, and more.)

The year 2022-23 is named '*Shubhkrut*', meaning 'that which creates auspiciousness.'

Most of the festivals in India are dated using this calendar. This calendar is unique because it is based on both the solar and lunar cycles. It indicates the phases of the moon and the location of the sun. Unlike the Gregorian month in the English calendar which has thirty or thirty one days, a Panchang month has fifteen tithis (dates) in each Paksha (fortnight) and each month is divided into two Pakshas.

While I was going through my cancer treatment, I rediscovered the importance of a value system and respect for every source of knowledge during the time I spent in solitude. However, proper human interaction and camaraderie are things that can be treasured for a long time. Honest relationships are becoming scarce. I consider myself very lucky and blessed to have the most caring people around me when I needed them the most.

It is also important to see situations from other people's perspectives. A biased opinion will always result in negative emotions. Having an open mind to discuss various issues from different angles is a desirable characteristic. At times, even a basic concept can offer the most demanding solutions.

I have mentioned some of the good habits that we must nurture and some that we should refrain from for the sanity of mind, body and soul.

> Speech is silver, but the silence is golden.

Other approaches in life may be responsible for inviting vicious diseases of the mind and body. Food is one that I have discussed earlier and so is hygiene. Sometimes out of haste, we resort to eating at places that might not be as hygienic as they should have been. We must not compromise our health and wellness for any reason. Hence, we should be taking more care about what and where we eat.

There is a famous saying, "Speech is silver, but silence is golden." In our day-to-day life, we always face situations where arguments meet anger and we tend to say words that we normally do not say and regret later. A seed grows with no sound, but a tree falls with huge noise. Destruction has noise, but the creation is quiet. This is the power of silence. It is always better to grow silently and keep a calm mind for the sake of our health and tranquility.

Despite having no vices, why did I develop cancer? This is a question that pops up in my mind very often. There is no clear answer to it. However, I feel that God wanted me to learn a few lessons and had chosen me to spread these teachings to other people too.

SAILING TO HEALTH

Good health does indeed have a profound effect on our well-being. It is also a fact that the best way to improve our well-being is to improve our physical, mental and psychological health. People who have good emotional control have fewer negative emotions and can bounce back from difficulties faster than others.

I understand that human life is full of surprises and at times it throws difficult challenges to test and measure the ability to be resilient. I accepted the fact that I was chosen to be tested for my resilience and mental strength with the challenges in my life. I responded to it with calm and composure and was treated with the most potent drug that can be administered for cancer. I was lucky that the cancer was detected at an early stage. This helped in my treatment and subsequent recovery.

Apart from the early detection and best treatment, I firmly believe that there are other aspects that worked in my favour. They helped me overcome the challenges and are important to know for the readers.

Hope

Hope is the greatest elixir for survival. I remember a famous line from the world-renowned peace activist and author, Thich Nhat Hanh, "Hope is important because it can make the present moment less difficult to bear. If we believe that tomorrow will be better, we can bear a hardship today."

During and after each of my chemo sessions, I often wondered whether I would be able to return to the thick of things. I missed my office routines and the various initiatives we had planned to implement. However, even during times when situations seemed uncontrollable, I held on to the hope that I would come out of this nightmare with more life lessons and surely be more enlightened.

Hope keeps one alive!

In India, cricket is like a religion. People are emotionally attached to the game in such a way that their behavior is heavily dependent on a win or loss for the country. In 2011, the Cricket World Cup was held in India. Many people had written off the chances of India winning the cup since no host nation had ever won it. India had somehow managed to reach the finals and was pitted against the strong team of Sri Lanka.

In the final match, Sri Lanka played first and managed to post a mammoth total on the board for India to chase in front of an over-excited home crowd. It was a huge challenge to achieve a big total under the lights, especially against a team with good-quality bowlers. India had lost their two legendary openers early on, which had brought gloom over a majority of the expectant spectators. However, the players and especially the captain did not lose hope.

India created history that night by scripting an epic victory that will forever remain embedded in cricket folklore.

Everything happened that night due to the hope, grit and hunger to win over seemingly insurmountable adversities. It was a learning lesson for me. Even if you are in a situation with your back against the wall, never lose hope. Fight on! If your intention and resolve are strong, victory cannot elude you—be it in cricket or cancer. People who succumb to unfortunate conditions tend to lose hope quickly.

Another aspect of life that keeps motivating me is to not fret about things that are not in our control. Even in religious scriptures, it has been written that we should always concentrate on things that are within our capability and the Universe will take care of the things that are not in our control.

In every phase of life, there are stumbling blocks and the hope that we carry sees us through to the other end. God must have better plans for each of us and we hope there will be positive results or conditions will ease the situation. The time will come when He will deliver but until then we should not lose hope and resort to recklessness. With strong hope, we can counter any misfortune in our lives. It is advisable to always be positive and have strong hope in our value system. Time rewards the hopeful.

Passion & Will Power

There is no doubt that there is no alternative to a passion and the will to make things better. I have always been passionate about engineering marvels. I have always been intrigued by how they could have been created centuries ago around the world when there was no computer, design software, sophisticated machines and not even too many trained engineers. There are a lot of such extraordinary examples of engineering marvels that still exist in the world. One such marvel that has amused me is the Brooklyn

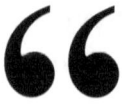

> With grit, passion and resilience, a bed ridden engineer who can not speak, has created an engineering marvel, 'The Brooklyn Bridge.'

Bridge, a landmark that tells the story of the passion and strong willpower of John Augustus Roebling and his son Washington Roebling, the master engineer who faced immense difficulties during the construction of this bridge. A bedridden engineer who could not speak led to the completion of the construction of a nearly impossible-looking one. Even after 140 years, the bridge is a testimony of great passion, the highest willpower and ultimate resilience.

When my test report came describing that I have a rare form of cancer, I felt my energy drain and thought that the report was overtaking my belief system. I summoned my willpower and there I was, telling my family members not to worry.

A strong will is a reflection of your passion and the positive attitude you carry. The inclination to go to any extent to derive a positive result is the outcome of a strong will. No matter the challenges, a determined person will always find ways to overcome them. Even during the most uncertain periods of my life, my strong will enabled me to endure the pain, fear, anxiety and unpredictability of my condition. The most important mantra had been the 'will to survive.'

It is a universal truth that humans are mortals and death is a reality that everyone must face at a particular time. However, the will to live is important to prosper rather than succumb to the first gust of wind. Despite knowing that we are all mortals, we still foster a fear of death. I have come to the realisation that I have a lot to do before my time comes to go. I didn't want to leave the world without achieving my dreams. I surely did not want to go bedridden in a hospital, overpowered by a disease.

I would rather move to the other world peacefully, having achieved my goals and in the presence of my loved ones. That was one of the motivations that kept away all negative possibilities. A strong will has made people stand out in a jostling crowd. The passion to make a difference and the will to live to do that are the main elements needed to sustain yourslef through tough and challenging times.

History is filled with stories about brave heroes who have overcome seemingly impossible situations to emerge victorious. The stories of Robert Bruce and Swami Vivekananda are great examples. Even people like Nelson Mandela or Mother Teresa had such strong wills. I had seen glimpses of this strong will in the eyes of people who had been there in strong support of me. My mother, wife, children, brothers, and close relatives always believed that I will come out unharmed. The power of their belief, faith and will gave me the necessary courage and strength to face my own challenges. We have seen athletes train for years to perform for just a few minutes in events like the Olympics. What keeps them going is their passion to win and their will to excel. It takes courage and a strong will to foster hope.

Food

Food is essentially any substance that living organisms ingest in order to sustain existence. We must be very careful and systematic in the selection of food items in order to properly nourish and benefit the body. Organic, unprocessed foods free from preservatives and chemicals are the best for the human body. Fried, deep-fried and packaged foods and sweets should be avoided as much as possible. In our religious books, it has been mentioned that one should always eat fresh, seasonal and local food. Just think about it: even 5000 years ago, junk food was derided.

It is also necessary to eat only when hungry. Pangs of hunger denote that the body has digested the food taken earlier and is craving more to supplicate the body with the necessary energy. Nowadays, a lot of food comes from warehouses and therefore, we get all types of food throughout the year. However, eating fresh seasonal fruits allows the body to accept them as the actual source of nourishment.

Additionally, milk is not a preferred food item. In fact, it is advisable to replace dairy milk with soy milk or almond milk and paneer and cheese with tofu. Seasonal fruit including watermelon and pineapple are good for the body and the digestive system. It is best to avoid packaged or canned food as they are full of preservatives.

Medicines also have some kind of side effects. Taking particular medicines frequently for small issues is not advisable because they merely suppress the symptoms for the time being although they have side effects that are sometimes more harmful.

Sometimes, our issues with food digestion and hyperacidity are acquired on our own due to not chewing our foods properly while eating. Most of us are always in haste while having food since it seems like an infringement on our schedules. Contrarily, eating the right way enhances our energy levels and boosts our immunity. What is the point of trying to save time by eating quickly if you are only going to lose more time to poor digestion levels and other illnesses? Food should be chewed, not gulped. Digestion begins in the mouth itself, and we should be mindful of this fact.

Fasting is a way of cleansing the internal organs. Intermittent fasting helps in re-organizing our system after the continuous onslaught of food that has to be processed by the various organs of the body. Fasting once a week or a month is not a great deal. In fact, all religions have advocated for fasting in some way or another. During some programs or festivals the body is under immense stress and hence, fasting a day before or after these events benefits the body by helping it recuperate.

> The Chinese and Japanese, who have a longer life span have the habit of drinking lukewarm water throughout the year, whatever the season might be. It is a practice that they have developed since time immemorial.

Water is an important part of our diet. Every dietician or doctor advocates for an adequate intake of water to keep the body hydrated and cool. However, we need to be careful about the water we drink. Not all bottled waters are healthy and suitable for our systems. It is advisable to have lukewarm water instead of cold water since the latter affects our system adversely.

Laughter

There is a fact in the famous saying, "Laughter is the best medicine." It is a great way to relieve stress, but it also has immense health benefits. One of the most important benefits of laughter is its ability to reduce the risk of heart disease.

Laughter is the best form of medicine for the mind. It is said that a day without laughter is a day wasted. Laughter sustains good hormones in the body and keeps negativity at bay. In many cities, laughter clubs have been set up to keep this healthy practice alive. It is no doubt that television shows that bring about laughter become hugely popular. We need laughter in our day-to-day lives. A simple session of laughter might act as the biggest stress buster for people.

During my treatment and subsequent recovery, I had been indulging myself in small laughter sessions with people around me. Small sessions of jokes or funny anecdotes worked wonders for the mind, and I always felt positive after every session. A cheerful face always emanates positivity. Even a cheerful refusal of an offer is accepted without much disappointment. A positive atmosphere can be fostered by keeping a cheerful attitude.

With so much power to heal and renew, the ability to laugh easily and frequently is a tremendous source for solving problems, enhancing relationships and supporting both physical and emotional well-being. The greatest fact is that this priceless medicine is fun, free, and easy to apply. It is also highly contagious. In an atmosphere filled with humour, it is difficult to stay gloomy.

Gratitude

Being thankful is a great attribute. We should be thankful for the little blessings we receive every day. How many of us thank our wives or mothers for cooking a delightful lunch or dinner? But this simple act goes a long way in brightening up their lives. Thankfulness is something that benefits both the giver and the receiver. Even small things are liable for gratitude. It is true that every employee in every domain receives monetary compensation for their services but an acknowledgement of gratitude brings about a spring in their steps. It doesn't cost anything but at the same time, it cannot be equated to money. We are thankful to be here as humans, enjoying the countless blessings of an ever-uncomplaining nature.

Being thankful is a great way to make life better. I could definitely say that the benefits I received in my life came from having an attitude of gratitude.

- Gratitude helps relieve stress.
- Gratitude makes you more positive.
- Gratitude strengthens relationships.
- Gratitude makes you healthier.
- Gratitude reduces the risk of depression.

- Gratitude is an affirmation of blessings and goodness that helps nurture a positive mindset and foster contentment.
- Gratitude is being thankful for the gift of life.

Expressing gratitude is another way of making people know that their efforts are being recognized. People need to feel appreciated and expressing gratitude helps people meet this need.

Kristin Armstrong, a professional road bicycle racer and multiple Olympic gold medalist has beautifully said, "When we focus on our gratitude, the tide of disappointment goes out, and the tide of love rushes in."

Importance of Good Sleep

Sleep is the greatest form of relaxation. During deep sleep, our organs have time to reorganize and revitalize. Sleeping and waking up at the right time is the highest form of healthy discipline. The recommended amount of sleep helps the body keep moving and avoid illness.

Therefore, it is advisable to relax thoroughly before getting to sleep. A timely and light dinner, listening to soothing music or indulging in some reading or breathing exercises before going to sleep is a good practice. Prayers and words of gratitude relax the mind. A good and sound night's sleep is equivalent to all immunity boosters put together. A stressful mind often disturbs sleep patterns. Try to wring out the stress before going to sleep. I have developed a habit of saying thanks to and showing gratitude by smiling at people around me. I also do it every night before retiring to bed for my family members even to my grandchildren who are too young to understand the meaning of it.

I would say from experience that adequate sleep has helped me maintain a good heart, keep my weight at the optimum level, have a sound mind and live stress-free.

A good night's sleep is vital for our health. In fact, it's just as important as eating a balanced, nutritious diet and exercising. We should also have set times to go to sleep at night. Staying awake late at night with mobile phones in our hands or watching television does not augur well for our bodies. Rather than staying up late, getting up early and doing our work or studies is more advisable.

Most adults require between 7 to 9 hours of good sleep every night. Yet, a high percentage of adults around the world don't get enough sleep or follow disturbed sleep patterns. Sleep deprivation can put our health at risk and therefore, we need to prioritize and follow a strict sleeping regimen.

Mentioned below are the reasons why we should not compromise our sleep patterns:

- Sleeping helps us maintain a proper body weight
- Good sleep improves concentration and productivity
- Good sleep maximizes physical and mental performance
- Good sleep helps to strengthen the heart and other organs
- Poor sleep causes mental disturbances like depression
- Proper sleep supports a healthy immune system
- Lack of proper sleep often causes increased inflammation
- Loss of sleep affects emotions and social interactions

Sleep helps us become more social and active. As a result, it can help us improve relationships. If you deal with loneliness or emotional outbursts, don't be afraid to reach out to a friend, family member, or healthcare professional to get support.

Forgiveness

Forgiveness is another attribute that has an immense influence on well-being. In circumstances where you might have been wronged or harmed, there is a possibility of having resentment, anger, disappointment, or regret for people and circumstances. However, if we hold a grudge and keep fostering feelings of resentment and vengeance, we tend to cause harm to ourselves. To keep our heads light and pure, we need to forgive all wrongs of the past and move on. By forgiving, I don't mean that we should support any wrongdoing but we should not delve into negative thoughts.

As the monk, Nithya Shanti, has said it is worth forgiving and forgetting the darkness in our past because there is light ahead.

"Sometimes it is worth to forgive and forget the past darkness because there is light ahead."

The capability of forgiveness is a virtue and it is for the welfare of our health and mental peace. The celebrated coach of TOC (Theory of Constraints), Eliyahu M

Goldratt, once said that there is no good or evil in the world and that people are driven by circumstances. Taking a cue from it, I suggest that we not let the circumstances overwhelm us. At the same time, people who do get influenced by the circumstances and resort to harmful activities should be avoided. Whenever a negative thought comes to mind, one must take at least 3 deep breaths and replace the thought with something relaxing like a happy incident from the past. As I said before, it is essential to keep a cool, composed and positive mind to stay healthy. By doing so, we can also curb the negativity that is prevalent in the world.

Patience

The world desires speed. The expectation is prevalent in all walks of life and gives rise to an ever-increasing emotion of impatience. We should realise that every activity cannot be done swiftly. There are many activities that are worth waiting for and making full use of it. I have seen people get frustrated due to things that do not happen as per their expectations. Remember that everything falls into place in due course, and the universe has specific plans for each one of us. Patience is a virtue of the mind.

The ability to wait for a result is indeed very taxing but once the wait is over, we are rewarded with happiness. Some of us think that they should be served first because of their position and stature in society but God treats everyone equally, so waiting for one's turn often brings better results in the end. We appreciate the patience of the doctors, nurses and caregivers because they boost our confidence when we are sick. A lot of patience is exhibited by our family members when they face problems. By being impatient and hasty, we often make the wrong decisions or commit a mistake that turns out to be harmful. If we can inculcate the habit of patience in our system, we can help our minds stay calm and positive.

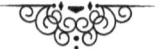

SOLITUDE CONNECTS YOU WITH YOURSELF

During my treatment and chemo sessions, there were moments when I found myself alone and I sensed that life was leading me instead of me leading my own life. I realized that in the fast-paced life that I was living so far, my life was controlled by numerous work schedules, demands, commitments, meetings, etc. Technology played a dominant role in ensuring constant connectivity through various means like emails, WhatsApp, social media, television, and even during commutes, where mobile phones were extensively utilized.

During the days I spent in solitude, I realized that there are aspects of life that we keep missing and during a particular stage of life re-discover the same with new flavors. I learned a lot of things that I had missed in my life during the stage of recovery when I had enough time to spend with myself. I find myself pondering how many of us can accurately determine the number of petals adorning a rose, the optimal moment in a spring morning when flowers emit their most delightful fragrance, and whether "Petrichor" (the scent of earth after rain) carries a sweeter aroma in the morning or the evening. There are a number of things we miss out on during our rush until we are halted by nature to have a look.

My adventurous nature has always made me push myself beyond my limits. I have always tried to not miss the joy that life presents us during the short stay that we are destined to spend on this planet. Still, there was much more to learn and during the time of recovery, I could devote time to these wonders and discover joy in every moment. However, there is still much to unravel. One lifetime is not enough to discover all the mysteries.

I highly recommend taking a pause in life. Take a moment to observe your surroundings, to observe yourself, to express gratitude for what you have; upgrade your thinking process, to look beyond your windows and observe nature—look at how the birds and animals conduct themselves—or to take a walk in nature.

I have always been enthralled by the sight of small saplings growing out of concrete pavements, brick walls, or the extensions of fallen trees. The will to live is inherent. It is a pity that we humans easily give up when we get interrupted by various circumstances. I have always believed that if the internal design of a system is stronger than the external barriers, the result will always be vibrant and full of life. Roses bloom among the thorns, lotuses bloom in muddy waters and tiny plants sprout from rigid pavements. When the will to live and thrive becomes stronger than the challenges we face, life emerges victorious over adversity.

Right from the beginning of my business career, when we started to evolve from a small water pump sales unit to a major EPC company in the seemingly difficult terrain of the North East, we never got overwhelmed by the imposition of the circumstances. The will to outgrow the challenges had a deep-rooted presence in our psyche and we always survived and even flourished during tough times. During my ailment too, I never let the fear of cancer rule my senses.

The will was to live through it like the saplings that grow out of dead trees, establishing a new form of life through harsh and adverse conditions. Despite the prevailing uncertainty evident in the distressed expressions of my loved ones upon learning of my cancer diagnosis, I remained resolute in my determination to overcome any obstacle that came my way, never doubting my strong will to endure tough times. Fear of fear is more fearful than fear itself. Once we accept our circumstances and live out of the disillusionment of the world of denial, we foster hope and learn to cope with fear and pain.

I Am a Cancer Survivor

I have survived through torrid times of uncertainty and fear of the unknown. However, my primary aim has always been to stay positive and upbeat even through difficult stages. I did not want to see my family members agonized by my health issues and I tried in every possible way to keep them optimistic and cheerful. During this roller-coaster ride through unpredicted events, I gathered a lot of learning from life which I believe is my responsibility to spread among the people in the world.

The paramount condition of life is that it has to be lived, under every circumstance, to the fullest degree. One should not miss out on the opportunity that God has bestowed upon them with the utmost kindness. I have always put on a brave face in front of every formidable challenge. This was also a test that I wanted to pass through with flying colours. However, I was able to learn more than I had expected to and I will always be thankful to God, my family and friends for that.

During my journey of revival from cancer, I realized that every passing moment had taught me some lessons about being a better human being. One doesn't need to be infected by a deadly disease or go through some traumatic experience to rediscover the joy of living and transforming. There is enough learning available if one is keen to observe and inculcate it in life.

Listed below are some of the crucial learnings I have acquired throughout the different phases of cancer. These attributes are what contribute to a life that is pure, happy, and delightful.

The Joy of Companionship

Testing times in life bring about the true value of meaningful relationships. However, it is very important to identify the right people to spend your precious time with. Apart from family members and blood relations, only a few genuine associates stick through the thick and thin in life. There are many people we come across in life with whom we consider spending time. Is everyone worth your precious time? Think about it. Sincerity in a relationship is important for harmony and coexistence but identifying the right kind of people is equally important for an association.

Families are important for numerous reasons. The definition of family seems to change with time, but it usually includes a group of people related to each other. Like many healthy social relationships, strong bonds with family members can have great benefits for society as well.

Family Improves Overall Well-being

Staying close to the family will benefit you in terms of physical health and happiness. After a thorough study, researchers have found that individuals who valued family and friends and developed important bonds and connections with them experienced better health throughout their lives. Staying isolated can increase a person's chances of distress and declining health. Family ties have been shown to provide stress relief by boosting self-esteem and reducing anxiety, especially for young people who have been exposed to violence. This strong bond can act as a protective shield and offer a sense of belonging during troubling times.

Elders in the family often act as the guiding stars. Young members look up to their elders and try to emulate them. Therefore, it is indeed a great responsibility of the elders to inculcate good habits in youngsters. When the older and younger generations in a family have strong bonds, it creates a close-knit unit that supports each other through tough times.

The kids in a family are great stress-busters. Their innocence and unadulterated emotions bring happiness to the family. A stressful day often melts into happy hours in the company of children. Children who experience healthy family relationships from an early age have better control over their emotions when they grow up. People who have more control over regulating their emotions are more self-aware and capable of dealing with tough situations appropriately and healthily. It is good to have elders as well as children in a family.

Family Helps Increase Lifespan

Researchers found that people without close relationships with family members other than a spouse were about twice as likely to die early in comparison to people with close family relationships. Strong familial connections surpass friendships in terms of their positive impact on longevity and overall well-being. There's something special about family members that makes people feel supported and happy.

Positive Feelings Help the Healing Process

In life, it is important to acquire the temperament of 'letting go.' There are people with negative viewpoints, an egoistic nature and selfish acumen in every society. It is important to identify them and try not to be in their company for long. We should practice the virtue of 'letting go' of associations that give us mental and emotional stress. All companionships and relationships should be meaningful and memorable. Life is short, and every moment is precious; therefore, the time that we spend with people should hold the right values and virtues.

Negativity has a huge bearing on our body system. Our nervous system, circulatory system and immune system are somehow connected to our paradigm of belief and when negativity enters our system, we tend to allow the ingress of diseases. The only method to safeguard against the unwanted access of disease or ill-conceived thoughts is to 'let go'.

Steve Maraboli has said, "Letting go means to come to the realization that some people are a part of your history, but not a part of your destiny."

Virtue of Acceptance

There are times in our lives when we live in a sense of denial, especially when the times are tough. It is common to blame circumstances, luck, people, governments or even God during testing times. However, acceptance of circumstances makes our life more peaceful and uncomplicated. By blaming others for our affairs, we generally end up intensifying our situation. Accepting the truth is a verity that provides both reasons and methods to sail through rough weather.

Upon learning about my cancer diagnosis, some individuals raised questions regarding how I could have developed it despite maintaining a healthy lifestyle. However, I did not waste my time on thoughts of denial. Instead, I concentrated on keeping myself upbeat and prepared myself for the battle against it. I believe that unpredictable situations come to those who can withstand, fight and overcome them. Weak people are not meant for challenges. Instead of asking "Why me?", one should be confident enough to say "Try me."

The virtue of acceptance is necessary to drive out the negativity of the mind and assert the feelings of resilience and grit to tame the bull by its horns. No challenge is terminal, even if it is cancer or COVID. With the proper mindset and acceptance of circumstances, one can effectively navigate challenges and setbacks and evolve in life.

Virtue of Kindness

One of the greatest virtues of life is being kind and considerate to everyone—not only to living beings but to everything. They might be inanimate, but they also deserve kindness. At times, when we get overwhelmed by circumstances, we tend to take things for granted. The food we eat, the air we breathe, the water we drink, the bed we sleep in, electricity, sunshine, rain, a cool breeze, greenery, relatives, friends, pets, clothes and many other things. It is during moments of crisis that we feel the importance of blessings that we otherwise do not notice. Acknowledge the importance of the various blessings that we get every day. The realization that we are surrounded by such essential amenities is the first step to bring happiness to our lives.

> Life is full of blessings; sometimes we don't value it.

Shakespeare once said, "I cried when I had no shoes, but I stopped crying when I saw a man without legs. Life is full of blessings, sometimes we don't value it."

What a meaningful line Anne Marie Cline has said: Today is the tomorrow that you dreamt about yesterday. This seems apt in the context of the present time. In our present time, we often find ourselves chasing after a better future, only to forget that we've longed for this very moment. Even if we remember, it's momentary. We immediately switch to thoughts about our upcoming future, attempting to attain more and more. Well, of course, we should always work hard and smart to do bigger and better things in life but, unfortunately, we often forget to cherish what we have already achieved. I would like to share an anecdote to reiterate this point.

One day, a king told his queen that on that day he would make the first person he saw when he stepped out of the palace happy. So, he found a beggar outside the palace and thought it would be so easy to make him happy. He gave the beggar a bag full of steel coins. While giving the bag, a few coins fell into the nearby gutter. So, the beggar kept the bag outside the gutter and started searching for the coins in the gutter.

The king thought that the beggar was not happy and hence, gave him a bag of silver coins. The beggar kept the silver coins outside the gutter and started searching again for those steel coins in the gutter. The king once again thought that the beggar was not happy, and he gave him a bag of gold coins. The beggar kept the gold coins outside the gutter and resumed his search for those steel coins in the gutter.

In our lives, we often find ourselves constantly seeking what we don't have, rather than appreciating and enjoying what we already possess.

Somehow, even in the testing times of my life, I had a flame of hope and positivity alive in my heart. Although I was striving to keep it burning, which was not visible from outside, it did exist. Thankfully, that helped me find happiness in the small things in life. When this was combined with a sense of gratitude, it worked wonders. During that difficult phase of life, whenever I was alone, I used to dive into my own world while looking at my surroundings for inspiration from nature and its beauty. Every time I did that, I discovered certain things that I was not aware of or may not have noticed.

The greatest gift that one can have is the life itself. There are so many things that we normally miss out on while making a livelihood for ourselves, and when we realize later what we missed, we feel sorry. Being thankful for the little things in life makes life more fulfilling.

After undergoing chemotherapy, the immune system of a patient comes down drastically. During that time, it is recommended that he isolate himself from others as the body becomes susceptible to infections. I had also been put on a similar regimen of quarantine to be safe and unaffected.

The process of knowing life and acknowledging its blessings is endless. Every day, I kept discovering new blessings. Today, I'm content and not restless about any scenario. I am not worried about getting more or having less. Most importantly, I am not comparing myself with anyone anymore and am not going to do that ever. I cherish my feet, and while I do work on getting a pair of shoes, I am not crying for them. I am thankful, I am content and I am blessed.

Virtue of Resilience

I belong to the world, and everybody should feel the same. I have travelled extensively across continents, countries, and cities, meeting people and learning the goodness of humanity from various traditions and cultures. I have always felt a palpable similarity in human nature everywhere. The colour of skin, food, religious beliefs or traditions might be different but humans have hugely common emotions everywhere. Tears of joy, yearning for company, the silence of grief, and expressions of fear and hope are common for all. We are just another species that behaves and emotes the same way as others.

Perhaps the biggest virtue of all is the emotion of resilience. Being a resident of Kolkata, I have witnessed a panorama of emotions run through the city. Kolkata is weaved through threads of emotions, where resilience, perhaps, forms one of the strongest strands.

Apart from the glorious ethos of centuries and heritage treasures like the iconic Howrah Bridge, Victoria Memorial, and other timeless glories, Kolkata also has the powerful urge to display the resilience it was born with. When you take a ride from the airport to the heart of the city, you see it all. An observant eye will invariably capture the essence of the city through its colours. There are colours so red that you would like to touch them and colours so blue that they startle you and tend to burn the back of your eyes. And then, your car comes to a screeching halt to allow a passerby, who limps across the street, to look back at you, as if muttering through his muted lips, "I owe respect, I am a human–soul."

In this city, I have learned to live through slogans and intellectual debate. I have learned to understand the strength of art and literature, to fight silent battles, and to be resolute in my aspirations. In this city, I have learnt to stand up and be counted among the courageous who strive for positive change and progress. I have learnt to sharpen my skill of resilience against the onslaughts of contrasting emotions. I owe this city a part of my livelihood and I am thankful that it made me a part of it.

There are times when even the most powerful people are left at the mercy of fate. The COVID pandemic proved this. There had been casualties even in some of the most sophisticated families that had a world of facilities under their command. I have always believed that destiny plays a major role in shaping the future events of one's life, despite the fame, stature, wealth and other attributes of an individual. It is always better to accept the ways of destiny instead of living in denial.

"This cannot happen to me" is a fool's paradigm. We are too unassuming to question the ways of the universe. Though we are a part of it, we are too small a fraction making us incapable of unraveling the intricate workings of our destiny. I have always been strong under all circumstances but this period has made me emerge stronger than ever.

My learning during this time is so valuable that I wish to share it with my readers.

1. **Never relinquish hope**: I had never given up hope, even during the most testing times in my life. My hope has never wavered, whether it be during difficult projects or the anxious moments throughout the detection and treatment of cancer, I have never lost hope. The positivity has always brought about encouraging results. I would like to suggest that if anyone is going through tough times, hold on to hope. Greater results await you.

2. **Never lose faith in God**: From the older generations of my family, I have inherited a profound conviction that a strong faith in God grants us the additional strength and resilience needed to withstand and endure challenging circumstances. God always has greater plans for us, and having faith in Him brings out the best in us. Testing times do come, but the time

for reward also comes to the one who believes and fosters the patience to wait.

3. **Spending meaningful time with family:** This is also another trait ingrained in me by my elders. Our family is our biggest asset and strength. I realized the importance of blood relations and family bonding during my difficult days when my wife, my sons, daughter, brothers, sisters and grandkids always tried to provide me comfort—the solace one requires during the testing times. It is our family that stands through thick and thin.

   Therefore, no matter how busy we may be, we should spend quality time with them regularly. By doing so, we are celebrating one of the greatest gifts of God. Take some time out of your busy schedule to spend with family. Those who are staying away from family/parents should connect by phone. The presence of family brings peace to one's mind.

4. **Do not give advice unless asked for:** It is never wise to advise anyone unless they ask for it. Unsolicited advice often creates annoyance. People always do their best when in trouble. By unnecessarily trying to guide people, one might upset their own plans for redemption. Even after my recovery from cancer, I never tried to impose my thoughts and experiences on people undergoing treatment. My elder daughter-in-law's mother too was diagnosed with cancer. Though I have talked to her several times, I have only tried to boost her spirits and never provided her with any unsolicited advice.

5. **Conquer your fears:** Generally, opinions cause anxiety and fear. I realized very early in my life that the worst fear is the fear of fear. We tend to imagine many things, even things that are exaggerated and unrealistic, by getting influenced by the fear

induced by unwarranted opinions. From a young age, I learned that fearlessness doesn't entail the absence of fear, but rather having reduced fear and, most importantly, possessing the attitude and desire to overcome it and improve circumstances.

The Real Pursuit of Life

I believe that the real pursuit of life should be happiness. Once we create different landmarks for ourselves, we get into a relentless rush to achieve them. Smaller things in life tend to get overlooked and ignored. The sunshine after a rainfall fails to make us happy. A good night's sleep fails to deserve the fulfillment it deserves. Homemade delicacies fail to attract our appreciation and thus, we miss out on the little happy moments that life presents us with every day. Probably, a sense of the concocted value of materialism has numbed our senses and we tend to equate materialistic acquisitions with the parameter of happiness.

In this context, I would like to tell you one interesting story that I heard during my schooling.

Despite the abundance of goodness within the prosperous kingdom, the king perpetually remained unhappy. The royal coffers overflowed with gold, the agricultural yields grew year after year, the loyalty of the people remained strong and undiminished, and the family of the king remained happy and prosperous. The king's gloominess never declined even an iota.

Concerned about the king's mental state, the queen called numerous mental health professionals to the kingdom for an examination. Most of the practitioners failed to find any reason for the discontent of the king and thus, could not offer any remedy.

However, an old advisor suggested that if the king could wear the shirt of the happiest person in the kingdom for a day, his mood could change.

Soon, soldiers were out in every direction to locate the happiest person in the kingdom. After a thorough search, they came across a man who looked gleeful throughout the day. People in the neighborhood vouched that he had always been happy, and they had never seen him grumpy. Realizing that he might be the man they were looking for, the soldiers went ahead and knocked on his door.

"The King needs a shirt from you since it was advised that wearing a happy man's shirt would change his mood," one of the soldiers announced from outside.

"Sorry, I cannot give him a shirt," the man replied from inside.

"What? You have the audacity to disobey royal orders?" The soldiers shouted with unrestrained wrath.

"I cannot offer him a shirt because I don't have any," saying this, a bare-bodied man emerged from the door and stood smiling at the stupefied soldiers.

This story tells us that it is not necessary to have a materialistic life with amenities to be happy. Satisfaction and being content are states of mind that do not require worldly materials.

This is the learning that I picked up in my journey from a humble beginning to the pinnacle of the corporate world. Most of this learning had been reinforced during my period of recovery from cancer and the subsequent recovery sessions after chemotherapy.

I fully believe that a person is the master of his life, and it is he who can make it either unfulfilling or rewarding. I remember a line from A. A. Milne. He said, "Always remember you are braver than you believe, stronger than you seem, and smarter than you think."

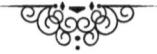

THE INSPIRATION

All my life, I have been inspired by great people from history and my contemporaries. My biggest inspiration comes from Lord Mahavir, the epitome of non-violence who was the 24th Tirthankar of the Jain religion. In the 6th century BC, Lord Mahavir was born into a royal family, but he renounced the world at an early age to become a monk. He preached for 30 years, and with deep meditation, he achieved enlightenment. Though he was born with worldly comforts, they never attracted him. But at the age of thirty, he left his family and the royal household, gave up his worldly possessions, and became a monk in search of a solution to eliminate the pain, sorrow, and suffering of people.

He spent the next twelve and a half years in deep silence and meditation to conquer his desires, feelings, and attachments. He carefully avoided harming or annoying other living beings, including animals, birds, and plants. He was calm and peaceful against all unbearable hardships and was given the name 'Mahavir,' meaning 'brave and courageous.'

Lord Mahavir preached that right faith (*samyakdarshana*), right knowledge (*samyakgyan*), and right conduct (*samyakcharitra*) together are the real path to attaining the liberation from karmic matter in one's self.

At the heart of right conduct for Jains lie the following ten great vows, which are called Tattvarthsutra.

1. Supreme forgiveness (Uttam Chama)
2. Supreme humility (Uttam Mardav)
3. Supreme straightforwardness (Uttam Arjav)
4. Supreme truthfulness (Uttam Souch)
5. Supreme purity (Uttam Satya)
6. Supreme self-restraint (Uttam Sanyam)
7. Supreme penance (Uttam Tap)
8. Supreme renunciation (Uttam Tyag)
9. Supreme non-possessiveness (Uttam Aakichanya)
10. Supreme celibacy (Uttam Brahmacharya)

I would like to tell you that during the COVID period, when people were mentally, physically and emotionally in distress, I embarked on a project that involved creating a series of 10 short videos with positive messages and life lessons to help people cope with fear and anxiety and a general sense of uncertainty. The above-mentioned 10 great vows became the theme of these videos and when we circulated them, people liked them and responded by taking steps to care for themselves and their families and managing to deal with stressful situations. These videos are available on 'Zian Life' YouTube channel.

Both men and women are equal in terms of spiritual progress, according to Lord Mahavir. The lure of renunciation and liberation attracted women as well. Many women followed his path and renounced the world in search of ultimate truth and happiness.

THE INSPIRATION

Thus, the principles of Jainism, if properly understood in their right perspective and faithfully adhered to, will bring contentment and inner happiness in present life. In future lives, the soul will ascend to a higher spiritual level, attaining perfect enlightenment and reaching eternal bliss, thus ending the continuous cycle of birth and death. Our family has been devout Jains. The principles of Jainism are deeply seated in our hearts and souls. I have always strictly followed every life value of Jainism and it has given me not only great mental strength but also a feeling of love and respect for all living beings. For me, Jainism is not only a religion but a way of life.

Books are my best friend, and I always like to read whenever I get time. I may have read countless books on diverse topics from inspirational to business, management to mysteries and even science fiction, among others. I have read widely about Nelson Mandela and how he kept his hope and inspiration by regularly reciting the poem *Invictus* by William Ernest Henley. 'Invictus' is a Latin word meaning 'undefeated.' Words, whether written or spoken, hold great power. This powerful song's provided him solace throughout his 27-year imprisonment. I believe that no power can stop a man on a mission and I always tell this to our engineers working on challenging projects far from city limits.

"Today a reader, tomorrow a leader" is a quote commonly attributed to Margaret Fuller. It refers to the belief that people who regularly read develop themselves and become leaders. Leaders draw wisdom from the knowledge they have gained by reading books. They always have a trove of knowledge and wisdom that they rely on to move forward. This sets them apart from non-readers, who often rely on more limited sources of information such as their personal experience and perspective to make critical decisions. It reminds me of Jim Rohn's words, "Successful people have libraries. The rest have big-screen TVs."

I had the privilege of meeting Mother Teresa and was influenced by her ever-caring nature for everyone. She was truly a mother to all the residents of Kolkata. Her aura was incredible and magical. Her efforts transformed the city's residents into a loving and caring place. I truly love her idea of living a purposeful life. Her perspective on life has always inspired me to live purposefully, and I believe you would agree with me as well:

> "Life is an opportunity, benefit from it.
>
> Life is beauty, admire it.
>
> Life is a dream, realize it.
>
> Life is a challenge, meet it.
>
> Life is a duty, complete it.
>
> Life is a game, play it.
>
> Life is a promise, fulfill it.
>
> Life is sorrow, overcome it.
>
> Life is a song, sing it.
>
> Life is a struggle, accept it.
>
> Life is a tragedy, confront it.
>
> Life is an adventure, dare it.
>
> Life is luck, make it.

THE INSPIRATION

Life is too precious, do not destroy it.

Life is life, fight for it."

In business mentorship, I have always admired the doyen of Indian industry, the affable JRD Tata. I met him during a journey as we both got the seats next to each other on a flight. He was a simple man with great vision and exemplary leadership. He redefined the business mantra in India and has made Tata Companies famous today. He not only dreamed about new business but also made full efforts to accomplish difficult-looking tasks. I'm happy that Tata has finally regained ownership of Air India, which was originally started by him. He was indeed a trendsetter, and I too dream of making such a valuable contribution to our nation and the world in the water domain.

> Never lose hope and never give up; success will come calling.

From the core of my heart, I am a deeply religious person and the teachings of Gurudevshri Kanji Swami has influenced my life significantly. He was a great saint of the 20th century who revived the Digamber Jain sect in India with his powerful religious discourse. He started a new revolution in the perception and practice of Jainism, thereby putting thousands of people on the true path of salvation. His followers are not only in India but are spread across several continents.

I admire Dr. Sanjeev Godha Ji for his approach to the spiritual principles of Jainism and their practical application in daily life through the new-age methodology. I had been following him, but his untimely demise has created a big vacuum.

I also follow the discourse of Acharya Shri Vidyasagar Ji who is considered a great monk of the Jain community. At the age of 76, his energy and tapasya (deep meditation) are still unmatched. He has been a true source of inspiration for millions of people to create institutions across the world for the welfare of all living beings.

I also admire the crystal thoughts and significant contributions of Munishri Pramansagar Ji, for making religious traditions more practicable in life. He is the most revered disciple of Acharya Shri Vidyasagar Ji. Through his focused initiatives and sermons, he brought about a qualitative change in society and led a campaign to save Jain traditions.

I am greatly influenced by the preaching of Acharya Shri Vardhaman Sagar Ji. His blessings during my treatment period have done wonders for me.

As I told you earlier, a habit I have inculcated since my student life is reading books. I do not remember how many books I may have read so far, but I can definitely tell you that put together at my home and office, I must have more than one thousand books on almost all leading topics. Whenever I visit a new place or a new country, I search for rare and valuable books and buy them. When returning from any trip, my luggage will have a number of new books. It is also my habit to mark the pages and note them in my diary where I feel they can be referred to in the future. At least, for my grandchildren, I will gift them a wonderful library.

THE INSPIRATION

I remember J. K. Rowling, the famous author of the Harry Potter series and philanthropist saying, "If you don't like to read, you have not found the right book." I feel blessed that wherever I go, I try to find the right kind of books that can enhance my learning and knowledge.

I take inspiration from Gaur Gopal Das's discourse as well. He is an electrical engineer but left his well-paying job to impart spiritual and management knowledge to people. His clarity of speech and thoughts are absolutely mesmerizing. He has a distinctive way of explaining spirituality and connecting it with modern-day life. Through his energetic talks, practicality, logical reasoning and subtle form of humour, he has motivated a lot of people and especially the youth across the world.

I truly believe in his dictum, "Don't regret knowing the people who come into your life. Good people give you happiness. Bad people give you experience. The worst ones give you lessons and the best people give you memories." I love meeting people and whenever I travel abroad, I make it a point to meet the native residents of that country, understand their culture, and way of life. I have always found inspiration from different cultures.

A spiritual teacher, and an exponent of Siddha Yoga, Swami Muktananda, has guided millions of followers in their spiritual development. He taught the traditional mystical doctrine of sadhana (spiritual discipline) and enhanced the ability of a person to awaken spiritual force through it. He authored many books and established over 600 meditation centers across the world to help spiritual seekers. I take inspiration from his sayings, especially his idea of loving yourself and your family.

He says, "The world is nothing but a school of love; our relationships with our husband or wife, with our children and parents, with our friends and relatives are the university in which we are meant to learn what love and devotion truly are."

I have discussed the importance of family, parents, children, and true friends in this book in several places. As I have said earlier, I take inspiration from great personalities and learn from them how to make life more fulfilling and joyful.

The attitude of never giving up does help in building a strong personality. When I was diagnosed with cancer, the initial thoughts that came to mind were fear and anxiety. But having a never giving up attitude, I recalled the words of Swami Gyanvatsal, a great saint and motivational speaker.

He says, "The moment you start giving reactions, and responses to negatives, you have accepted negatives in life." This thought has given me immense strength and courage to confront the challenges I've encountered. I'm grateful to God for accepting the challenge and successfully overcoming it. I regularly hear his motivational talks, and believe me, the way he describes life's difficult challenges and how to deal with them is really inspiring.

There are many great achievers in history and present times from whom one can learn. Every day, I make it a habit to listen to motivational and spiritual leaders. Often, I carry my

My father was an upright man with strong passion for life.

diary with me to jot down the beautiful and important points they share. I would suggest that we inculcate the habit of listening to and following such personalities for the tranquility of mind and soul.

Whenever I come to know about any personality, I always ensure that I read their stories, autobiographies, etc. and take inspiration from them.

It would be incomplete, if I did not mention my beloved father, Punam Chand Sethi ji whose tremendous influence is visible in my life. Both of my brothers and I got trained to manage the business under his supreme guidance and able leadership. We acquired humility from him and developed a never-say-die attitude as a result of his example. He has instilled in us confidence and courage while giving us the freedom to explore, take risks and learn practical life lessons. While talking about him, I can go on and on but one thing I am sure that my brothers will also agree with me that his soft nature, ethical values and exceptional way of parenting has helped us foster empathy, honesty, courage, and self-reliance. I will always be thankful to God for blessing us with such a great man and a great parent.

I strongly believe that when individuals give their best, utilizing their skills and expertise, and willingly share their knowledge and experiences, it will greatly benefit humanity by harnessing the virtues inherent in each person. God has blessed every person with diverse knowledge and extraordinary capabilities.

It's true that people should make an effort to share knowledge, experiences, and values with others. By doing so, we can help them become more knowledgeable and capable of making informed decisions. This, in turn, contributes to creating a better world to live in.

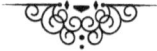

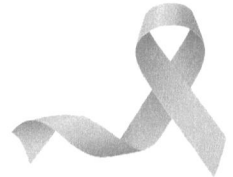

MY HEARTFELT MESSAGE

An inspirational quote from Amanda Gorman that has touched my heart: "There is always light. If only we were brave enough to see it. If only we are brave enough to be it." I firmly believe that we should have a vision to see that light and be guided in life.

Besides becoming a cancer survivor, I am also fortunate to have learned a lot about life that I wish to share with the world. It has been a painful process of learning. Yet, I am thankful to God for having allowed me to gain these insights. My mission in business is continue to contribute glorified feathers to the magnificent cap of the company, SPML Infra Limited, enhancing its illustrious reputation and adding to the impressive laurels we have already achieved. We aspire to become a globally acclaimed company in water management with sustainable business growth. Professionally, I will ensure that our company keeps on scaling greater heights and it becomes the most admirable company among its peers.

I want to personally discover lesser-known places in our country that have beautiful natural scenery and a peaceful ambiance, allowing me to connect with nature. As a member of the Indian Cancer Society, I would like to contribute more to society and our country.

I would like to be a part of other cancer societies to spread awareness about this disease and help patients cope with it in a dignified way.

> I aspire to make positive contributions to people's lives through innovative and novel initiatives and inspire them to think beyond their limits and achieve the unthinkable. The only way to make a country great is if every citizen thinks and acts in a complementary manner.

The contents of this book are based on my personal experiences and what I learned while going through cancer treatment and recovery. Some people might be suffering from various stages of this disease. Cancer is now fully curable if detected at an early stage of infection. Therefore, one should not ignore any persistent ailment. Additionally, it is always advisable to get several opinions before going for any vigorous treatment.

It is also important to note that the reactions, communications, and body language of the doctors and other medical staff contribute greatly to the recovery of a patient. It is a very sensitive disease. So, breaking the news to the patient and family has to be done with concern and empathy. Delivering bad news improperly may devastate a family. During treatment, we must keep in mind that the situation is maintained with a positive spirit. With my experience of meeting several doctors in different cities, I highly recommend that doctors and other medical professionals give their undivided attention to the patients, and listen to them carefully and with genuine concern and clearly explain the steps of treatment and potential outcomes.

Above all, one should have a deep belief in God to ensure the success of treatment. I do not intend to profess any particular form to be worshipped or prayed to. Whatever form evokes a sense of devotion and faith can be used to believe. A complete feeling of serendipity bolsters the hope from within.

I would also suggest that a patient stay close to family. Being with your loved ones gives you the internal strength to fight any adversity.

Be careful when choosing your friends. Toxic people may poison your mind and fair-weather friends do not stick around for long. During tough times, you will find your family and only true friends will remain by your side.

The environment today is full of negativity. However, if one can hold on to positive thoughts and be grateful for even the little things in life, good outcomes are bound to happen. I believe that this disease or any other serious ailment can be effectively combated with the right combination of medical treatment and mental strength. At no time, should one let negativity encircle the mind. Reminding ourselves of the countless blessings God has bestowed upon us and cherishing them creates an aura of positivity. It is also necessary to celebrate even small occasions and achievements with the family. These little joys are indeed priceless and bring the family much closer.

Hope is something that acts as a catalyst for recovery in all difficult situations. However, to have an effective recovery one must also be careful about the food being consumed. I have described in the earlier chapters, sweets and fried food have adverse effects on health and encourage harmful cells to grow, including cancer cells. To stay healthy, it's best to prevent cancer cells from getting nourishment.

Today, after having recovered from cancer, I believe that there is a greater calling for me to make a better contribution to society. God has willfully granted me this opportunity to use my learning and resources for the greater good. I feel thankful and blessed to be chosen for that.

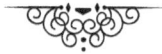

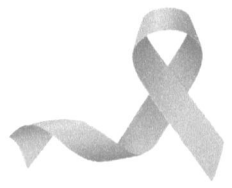

THE VIEWPOINTS

There are some quotations and observations that help us understand cancer from the doctors or survivors' points of view and enrich our knowledge. I would like to share some of them here which are informative and encourage you to fight the demon and not surrender to it.

"You can be a victim of cancer or a survivor of cancer. It's a mindset."

– **Dave Pelzer**

"I am not afraid of storms, for I am learning how to sail my ship."

– **Louisa May Alcott**

"Before I started chemotherapy treatments, I wrote down the best advice from doctors, family, friends, books, and survivors and created an 'Owner's Manual' to help me take care of myself. It would remind me that cancer is doable."

– **Regina Brett**

"As a cancer doctor, I'm looking forward to being out of a job."

– Daniel Kraft

"Today is my day! Wish you all a happy #worldcancerday and hope each one of us celebrates this day in an embracing way. That we remove any stigma or taboo associated with it. That we spread awareness about it and that we have self-love, no matter what. I truly embrace all my scars, as they are my badges of honour. There is nothing known as perfect. Happiness lies in truly accepting yourself. This was a tough one for me."

– Tahira Kashyap Khurrana, Cancer Survivor

"Cancer has taught me a lot of things. Maybe it is the best thing that has happened to me. I can't say right now, but maybe some years down the line, I would realise. When I was undergoing chemotherapy, there were a lot of elderly patients, and that would inspire me. I thought, 'If they can be cured, why can't I be?'"

– Yuvraj Singh, Cricketer and Cancer Survivor

"Cancer became my teacher. It taught me to seek out help in various aspects influencing my health. It led me to learn yoga and pranayama, and encouraged me to deepen my spiritual understanding by going to Oneness University."

– Manisha Koirala, Bollywood Actress and Cancer Survivor

THE VIEWPOINTS

"The first step to fight cancer is to be happy. I feel when it comes to fighting cancer, 50 percent cure can be attributed to medication and another 50 percent to willpower."

— **Anurag Basu, Bollywod Film Director and Cancer Survivor**

"Cancer has shown me what family is. It showed me a love that I never knew really existed."

— **Michael Douglas, Hollywood Actor and Cancer Survivor**

"In 2005, a man diagnosed with multiple myeloma asked me if he would be alive to watch his daughter graduate from high school in a few months. In 2009, bound to a wheelchair, he watched his daughter graduate from college. The wheelchair had nothing to do with his cancer. The man had fallen down while coaching his youngest son's baseball team."

— **Siddhartha Mukherjee, (Indian-American physician, biologist, oncologist, and author)**

"If you want to change something, you need to keep walking, progressing. Amidst this, there will be successes and failures. But, as long as the intention is good, things will happen. You just need to keep walking."

— **Dr. Devi Prasad Shetty, Philanthropist, Cardiac Surgeon, Padma Bhushan Awardee**

"Don't let pain define you, let it refine you."

– Tim Fargo

"Pain is temporary, it may last a minute, or an hour, or a day, or a year, but eventually it will subside and something else will take its place. If I quit, however, it lasts forever."

– Lance Armstrong, World Cycling Legend and Cancer Survivor

"Cancer is a word, not a sentence."

– John Diamond

"As it turned out, everyone knew that I had cancer. That is, everyone except me."

– Brett M. Cordes, "Cancer is for Old(er) People: How Young Minds Beat an Old Disease"

"Believe in your prayers. Believe in the power of your faith and the blessings of your near and dear ones. Their love serves as a balm, soothes your heart and heals your body."

– Sanchita Pandey, Cancer to Cure

"Let's not call cancer patients as patients, they are cancer fighters. They are brave hearts."

– Vikram, Guru with Guitar

"There is beauty in finding the silver lining, even though the darkness. It is there if you search for it."

– Tracey Ehman

"Difficult roads can lead to beautiful destinations."

– Kia Wynn, Cancer Survivor

"I learned that courage was not the absence of fear, but the triumph over it. The brave man is not he who does not feel afraid, but he who conquers that fear."

– Nelson Mandela

"Look to this day for it is life. For yesterday is already a dream and tomorrow is only a vision. However, if today is well lived it makes every yesterday a dream of happiness, and every tomorrow a vision of hope."

– Sanskrit Proverb

"When the Japanese mend broken objects, they aggrandize the damage by filling the cracks with gold. They believe that when something's suffered damage and has a history, it becomes more beautiful."

– Barbara Bloom

"Cancer is that awful word we all fear when we go to the doctor for a physical exam, but in that brief dark moment we hear it the world we live in and the people we share it with begin to illuminate things we did not even pay attention to."

– B.D. Phillips

"Be strong, be fearless, be beautiful. And believe that anything is possible when you have the right there is a people there to support you."

– Misty Copeland

"It's possible not just to survive, but to thrive and to live a healthy, wonderful life again."

– Erika Evans, Cancer Survivor

"For every wound, scar, and every scar tells a story. A story that says, "I survived!""

– Craig Scott

"Always remember you are braver than you believe, stronger than you seem, smarter than you think and loved more than you know."

– Christopher Robin

"Don't count the days, make the days count."

– Muhammad Ali

"You are your own person—the only person that will go through this physically and you have every right to share and provide yourself with every ounce of control. Your voice is your power."

– **Nina L., Non-Hodgkin Lymphoma Cancer Survivor**

"There are many great doctors and nurses out there that are on your side and they're going to get you through it. It does get better."

– **Evan, Acute Lymphoblastic Lymphoma Cancer Survivor**

"What's in my control is taking care of myself and being healthy. I've found peace and solace in knowing I'm doing my part and I've found this in the fact that whatever will happen will happen."

– **Jason F., Hodgkin Lymphoma, Stage 2A Cancer Survivor**

"Life isn't about finding yourself. Life is about creating yourself."

– **George Bernard Shaw**

"Happiness is not something readymade. It comes from your own actions."

– **Dalai Lama**

"Believe you can and you're halfway there."

– **Theodore Roosevelt**

"Today I choose life. Every morning when I wake up I can choose joy, happiness, negativity, pain... To feel the freedom that comes from being able to continue to make mistakes s and choices—today I choose to feel life, not to deny my humanity but embrace it."

– **Kevyn Aucoin**

"Put your heart, mind, and soul into even your smallest acts. This is the secret of success."

– **Swami Sivananda**

"Thousands of candles can be lit from a single candle, and the life of the candle will not be shortened. Happiness never decreases by being shared."

– **The Buddha**

FREQUENTLY ASKED QUESTIONS (FAQS)*

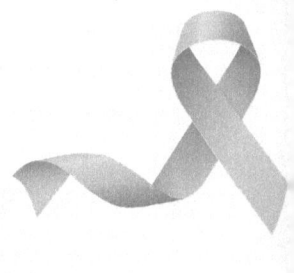

For decades, sometimes the simplest of questions about cancer have gone unasked or unanswered. It is therefore essential to understand the most common thoughts that involve cancer.

1. How can one get infected?

Anyone, at any age, can become infected by cancer, however the risk increases with age. There are individual risks too that depend upon factors such as smoking, eating unhealthy food, disorganized lifestyle, lack of exercise, family history of cancer, and other components related to stress, pollution and personal habits.

2. How does cancer take shape in the body?

The human body is made up of millions of various kinds of cells. Under normal conditions, cells grow, divide, become old, die and get replaced by new cells. However, in a few cases, cells mutate and grow out of control, and form a mass or tumor instead of following the regular regime of degeneration or dying.

Tumors can be benign (noncancerous) or malignant (cancerous). Cancerous tumors can attack and kill the tissues of the body. They

* Source: www.foxchase.org/blog

can also spread to other parts of the body, causing new tumors to grow in different areas. This process is called metastatic and it represents cancer that has progressed to an advanced stage.

3. Is cancer genetic?

It has been established that cancer has a genetic connection. This is due to the fact that cancer is produced by mutations or alteration to genes that control how our cells function, causing them to behave abnormally. These mutations can be inherited, as they are in about 5-10 percent of all cancer cases but it's much more likely that these changes in genes occur during a person's lifetime due to other factors besides genetics.

When someone has a known family history of hereditary cancer, genetic testing is often recommended.

4. Is cancer contagious?

No. Cancer isn't like the flu, viral fever or a cold. You can't catch cancer from someone who has the disease.

5. Is there a vaccine for cancer?

There is no vaccine for cancer. But there are vaccines for some viruses that are known to cause cancer, such as the human papillomavirus (HPV) and hepatitis B. HPV can cause cancer, and getting vaccinated against it can help protect against the types of HPV that can lead to cervical, anal, throat, and penile cancers, along with some other forms of cancer. The HPV vaccine protects against many strains of the virus that can cause these cancers.

THE VIEWPOINTS

The same is true for infection with the hepatitis B virus, which has been linked to liver cancer. Getting vaccinated against hepatitis B can reduce your risk of getting liver cancer. However, just like the HPV vaccine, the hepatitis B vaccine doesn't protect against liver cancer itself. It only protects against the virus that might lead to liver cancer.

6. Can cancer be cured?

Yes. Often we hear the doctors say that the cancer is in remission. A partial remission occurs when the cancer shrinks but doesn't disappear. Complete remission means there is no longer any sign of cancer. The longer a cancer is in complete remission, the less likely it is to come back, and at some point, doctors might say that the cancer has been cured.

7. What are the stages of cancer, and what do they mean?

Cancer typically has four stages: I through IV. Some cancers even have stage 0 (zero). Here's what these stages mean:

Stage 0: This stage means the cancer is still found in the place it started and hasn't spread to nearby tissues. Stage 0 cancers are readily curable.

Stage I: This stage usually represents a small tumor or a lump that hasn't grown deeply into nearby tissues. It's sometimes called early-stage cancer.

Stages II and III: Usually, these two stages represent the phase where larger tumors may have grown more deeply, spread into nearby tissues, and spread to lymph nodes and other areas too.

However, they wouldn't have spread to other organs or parts of the body.

Stage IV: During this stage, the disease spreads to other organs or parts of the body. It is often referred to as metastatic or advanced cancer.

8. Does cancer show some early symptoms?

In some cases, it does, but not always. The signs and symptoms of cancer depend on where the cancer is located and how big it is. As the cancer starts growing, it can push onto nearby organs and other structures of the body. The resulting pressure can cause signs and symptoms like pain and irritation.

Some types of cancer may grow in places where they do not show any signs or until they have reached an advanced level. For example, pancreatic cancer usually doesn't show any symptoms until it grows large enough to press onto other organs, causing pain or showing signs of jaundice, by bringing about yellow pigmentation in the skin.

Some general signs of cancer are common for all types:

- Unexplained weight loss
- Persistent fever
- Continuous feeling of fatigue
- Pain in certain areas
- Skin changes in texture and pigmentation
- Irregularity in bowel and bladder function
- Sores that remain even after medication
- Unusual bleeding or discharge

- A thickening or lump in a part of the body that doesn't diminish in size
- Indigestion or trouble swallowing food and fluids
- A change in the texture of a wart or mole in the body
- An irritating cough or hoarseness of voice

Of course, there can be other reasons for these symptoms. It is advisable to consult a doctor or even more than one doctor if such signs can be observed. These signals should never be ignored or neglected.

9. How do cancer drugs work?

Chemotherapy uses chemical concoctions to destroy cancer cells. Though chemotherapy may have side effects, it is still the most dependable treatment. The side effects generally reduce over time, if healthy lifestyle practices are resorted to.

New methods of treatment are also being used for various types of cancer, and a lot of research is being done presently to economize the treatment and make it readily available.

10. When should one get tested for cancer?

Regular medical tests are recommended so that any ambiguity in body function may be screened out. When there is some abnormal growth observed in any body part, immediate medical attention should be sought.

11. What are the most common forms of cancer?

- Blood Cancer
- Breast Cancer

- Lung Cancer
- Cervical Cancer
- Colorectal Cancer
- Oral Cancer

These are some of the commonest cancers of the present times.

12. Has the survival rate of cancer improved over the years?

Definitely! Cancer can be easily detected nowadays in its primary stages. Therefore, the cure for the disease is more result oriented causing the survival rate to increase with every passing year. There have been more cancer survivors in recent years in comparison to the earlier decade. Cancer is no longer as dreadful as it once was.

Some recommendations for common types of cancer:

Breast cancer

Global research has observed that women who undergo routine screening mammograms are more likely to have their breast cancer detected early and get cured.

It is therefore recommended that all women over the age of 35 undergo a formal risk assessment for breast cancer at some time during routine medical checkups.

For people at average risk for breast cancer:

- **Women 40 and older:** An annual mammogram is recommended during routine checkups at least once every 6 months.

Cervical cancer

Regular check-ups can easily detect cervical cancer in its earliest stages. Almost all cervical cancers are caused by the human papillomavirus (HPV) and most are asymptomatic in their early stages. Screening for HPV can find an infection that could ultimately lead to cervical cancer.

Colorectal cancer

These types of cancers develop from inflammation of the bowels and disorders in their functions. There are several types of tests to check for colorectal cancer. Stool tests and other such pathological investigations can determine the disease after it has reached a developed stage. Some tests like colonoscopy, can find both polyps (abnormal growths) and cancer. If polyps are found during investigations and tests they can be removed, reducing the risk of developing cancer in the future.

People who often have problems with bowel movements and inflammations are generally at risk for colorectal cancer and one should regularly take a doctor's advice after attaining the age of 45. Doctors can best advise which screening test is best for people and how often they should need it.

If for instance, you have a family history of colorectal cancer or a personal history of inflammatory bowel disease, you may need to start consulting a doctor before the age of 45 or be tested more often as per the advice of the doctors about your risks.

Lung cancer

Many people remain ignorant that they have lung cancer until symptoms appear, when the disease may have reached an advanced stage. In recent years, testing tools such as a low-dose CT scan have been developed that can help catch lung cancer in its early stages, when treatment can provide the best outcome.

The following criteria are often taken into consideration for the need for a low-dose CT scan, of course after consulting the doctors:

- You're between the ages of 50 and 80.
- You have a history of heavy smoking – for example, you have smoked the equivalent of a packet a day for 20 years, or you have been exposed to industrial gases/emissions, or automobile emissions for more than a decade.
- You still smoke, have quit within the last 10-15 years, or live near areas of heavy air pollution.

Skin cancer

The human skin is the largest organ in the body and also one of the most important defenses for the internal organs. Therefore, it is important to keep it properly guarded. Regular checking of the skin for changes in moles, marks or colour can help detect skin cancer early, particularly for people exposed to harsh environmental conditions.

A dermatologist's skin examination is always suggested on a regular basis. It is also advisable to examine your skin on your own once a month. Check your entire body, using a hand mirror for hard-to-see areas like your back and behind your ears. Even for a moment, do not hesitate to meet your doctor if you notice anything different about your moles, marks, or pigmentation.

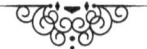

CANCER ETIQUETTE*

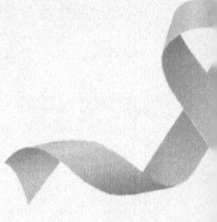

Cancer is no longer a silent disease.

It can be difficult to know what to say to someone with cancer. Unless you've been there yourself, you can't possibly understand how it feels.

Many people say inappropriate things without realizing it. We often do the best we can, but our efforts still fall short. How do we find the right words to talk to someone with cancer?

Years ago, people spoke in whispers about cancer. Today, despite its prevalence, advances in treatment, and increasing survival rates, many people still don't know how to handle the news.

At some point, someone you know will likely get cancer. When it happens, you should be prepared to communicate appropriately about the disease.

Numerous cancer patients and survivors have common experiences of uncomfortable encounters and disheartening remarks from even close family members. Their collective observations help us define 'cancer etiquette,' or rules of conduct for communicating with the cancer community. Since each person experiences cancer differently, one approach does not necessarily

*Source: www.cancercenter.com

work for everyone. This information serves as a starting point for talking to someone with cancer. There is no single right way. Just keep trying.

Tips for talking to someone with cancer

Don't ignore them. Some people disappear when someone they know gets cancer. The worst thing you can do is avoid the person because you don't know how to handle it. Cancer can be lonely and isolating as it is. Tell them, "I'm here for you," or "I love you, and we'll get through this together." It's even okay to say, "I don't know what to say," or send a note that says, "I'm thinking of you." Just stay connected.

Think before you speak. Your words and actions can be powerful. One comment can instantly undo someone's positive mood. Don't be overly grave and mournful. Avoid clichés, like "hero" and "battle." If the person gets worse, does it mean they didn't fight hard enough? Try to imagine yourself in your friend's shoes. What would you want someone to say you?

Follow their lead. Let the person with cancer set the tone for what he or she wants to talk about. It doesn't always have to be about cancer. Chances are your friend wants to feel as normal as possible. Tell him or her about something funny that happened. Allow your friend to talk about cancer if he or she wants. And do not have pitiful eyes or tone.

Keep it about your friend, not you. Don't lose your focus. Avoid talking about your headache, backache, etc. This isn't about you. And as bad as you feel, he or she feels worse and may not be interested in hearing about how hard this has been on your life.

Don't put him or her in the position of having to comfort you. Only ask questions if you truly want to hear the response.

Just listen. Sometimes just being there to listen—really listen— is the best thing you can do. Let the person with cancer talk without interrupting. You don't always have to have all the answers, just a sympathetic ear. He or she may not talk at all and would rather want to sit quietly. It's okay to sit in silence.

Don't minimize their experience. Try not to say, "Don't worry, you'll be fine." You don't know that. Instead say, "I'm really sorry," or "I hope it will be okay." And don't refer to his or her cancer as "good cancer." These statements downplay what he or she is going through. Leave the door to communication open so they can talk about their fears and concerns.

Don't be intrusive. Don't ask those with cancer questions about their numbers or tumor markers. If they want to talk about their blood results, they will. Give them the freedom to offer this information or not. Also, don't ask personal questions that you wouldn't have asked before, especially when it comes to subjects like sex and religion.

Don't preach to them. Don't try to tell the person with cancer what to think, feel or how to act. You don't know what they're going through, so don't act like you do. Instead of saying "I know how you feel," try saying "I care about you and want to help." Don't suggest alternative forms of treatment, a healthier lifestyle, etc. And don't tell them to "stay positive", it will only cause frustration and guilt.

Refrain from physical assessments. Refrain from making comments about how those with cancer look, particularly if they

CANCER ETIQUETTE*

are negative. They don't need their weight loss or hair loss pointed out to them. And if they just started treatment, don't ask them about potential side effects. If you say anything at all, tell them they look stronger or more beautiful, but mean what you say.

Avoid comparisons. Everyone deal with cancer in his or her own way. Don't bring up the private medical problems of other people you know. And don't talk about your friend with cancer who is running marathons or has never missed a day of work. Avoid talking about the odds or making assumptions about the prognosis. Just allow your friend to be who they are.

Show them you care. Show those with cancer that they're still needed and loved. Give them a hug. Surprise them with a smoothie, books, magazines, or music. Offer to help, such as with cooking, laundry, babysitting or running errands. Be specific by asking, "What day can I bring you dinner?" And, offer to help only if you intend to follow through with it and won't expect anything in return.

Share encouraging stories. Offer encouragement through the success stories of long-term cancer survivors. Avoid saying, "They had the same thing as you." No two cancers are alike. And never tell stories with unhappy endings. If you know someone with the same type of cancer, offer to connect the two of them.
Source: www.cancercenter.com

REFERENCES

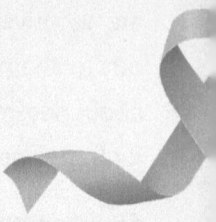

It is necessary to know some of the best doctors and hospitals in the country that could be consulted when confronted with cancer. This list is of those doctors with whom I consulted and got my treatment under their supervision. Only those hospitals are mentioned here where my medical investigation and treatment have taken place, these are of course not exhaustive, but important contacts that may help someone in need.

List of Doctors

Dr. Naresh Trehan Chairman & MD Medanta Hospital, Gurugram	naresh.trehan@medanta.org
Dr. Nitin Sood Director Hemato Oncology & Stem Cell Transplant Medanta Hospital, Gurugram	docnitinsood@yahoo.com

REFERENCES

Dr. Ashok Vaid Chairman Hemato Oncology Cancer Institute Medanta Hospital, Gurugram	dr.ashokvaid@indiacancersurgerysite.com
Dr. Deepak Sarin Vice Chairman Head and Neck Oncology Cancer Institute Medanta Hospital, Gurugram	deepak.sarin@medanta.org
Dr. Ankur Bahl Senior Director Medical Oncology & Hematology Fortis Memorial Research Institute, Gurugram	ankur.bahl@fortishealthcare.com
Dr. Anita Borges Lab Director Centre for Oncopathology Mumbai www.oncopath.org	info@oncopath.org
Mr. Luke Coutinho Nutritionist, Holistic & Wellness Coach	info@lukecoutinho.com

List of Hospitals

Medanta, The Medicity Hospital, Gurugram
www.medanta.org

Tata Memorial Hospital, Mumbai
www.tmc.gov.in/tmh

Fortis Healthcare Hospital
www.fortishealthcare.com

Max Super Specialty Hospital
www.maxhealthcare.in

Aakash Healthcare Hospital
www.aakashhealthcare.com

Mount Elizabeth Hospital, Singapore
www.parkwaycancercentre.com

Mayo Clinic, California, USA
www.mayoclinic.org

Apollo Hospital
www.apollohospitals.com

I N S P I R E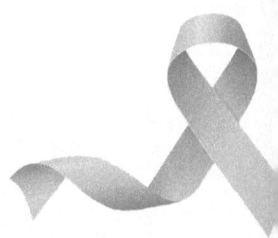

I nfuse positive energy and zest for life

N urture new ideas and visions

S ummarize complex concepts and ideologies

P rovide us with a new perspective of seeing things

I nspire us to have dreams

R eveal the mindset of successful people

E ncourage us in times of despair

This book contains my true story of fighting back cancer and my learning during the entire phase of treatment and recovery. I have thoughtfully incorporated handpicked quotations and verses from famous personalities in various chapters to remind us of our inner strengths and abilities to fight adversities in life. I do hope the empowering words in this book will inspire you to reach higher.

Thank you,

Subhash Sethi

www.ingramcontent.com/pod-product-compliance
Lightning Source LLC
LaVergne TN
LVHW041924070526
838199LV00051BA/2716